HOMESTYLE MEDITERRANEAN

Rustic Cooking from Around the Sea

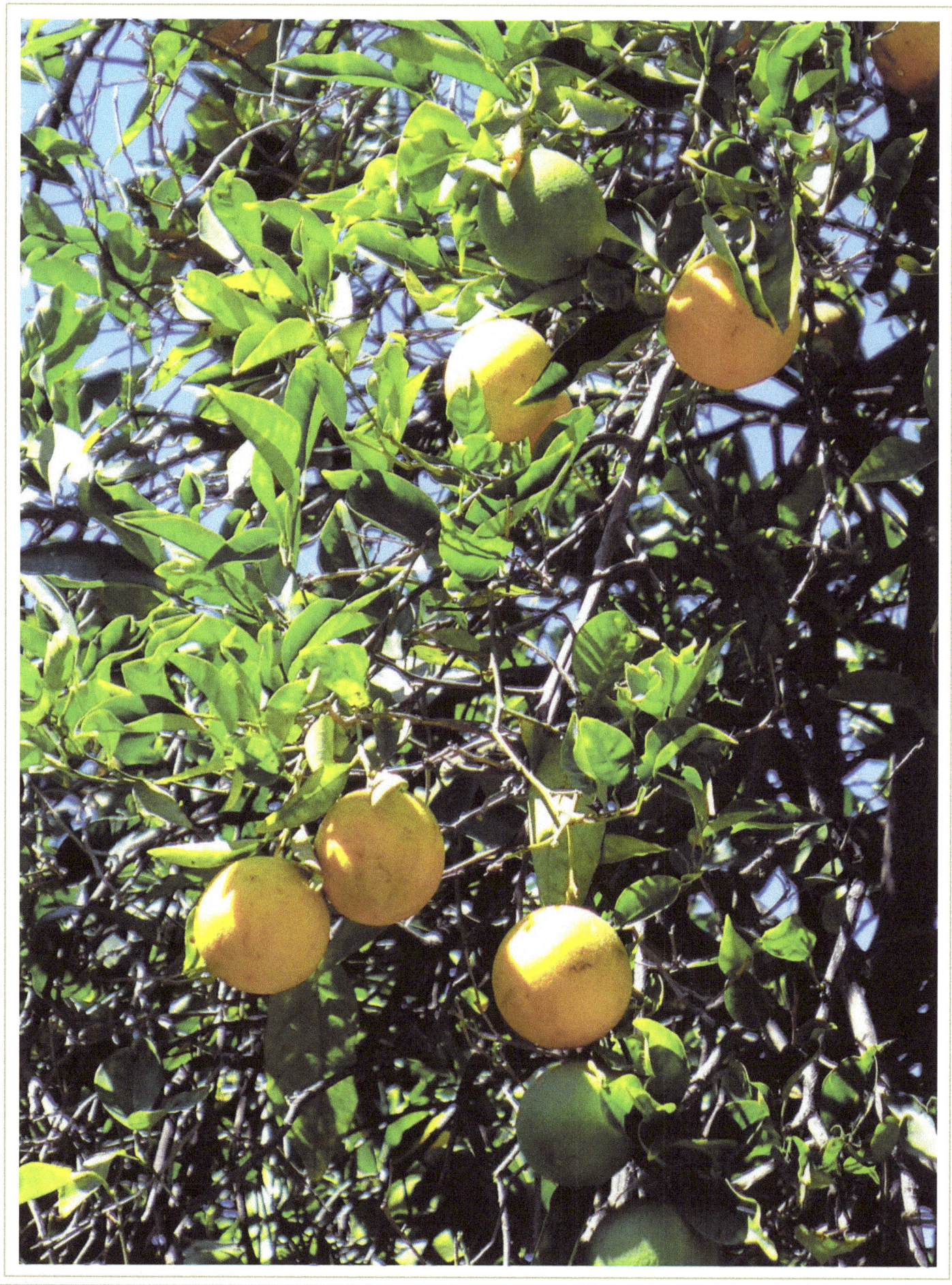

HOMESTYLE MEDITERRANEAN

Rustic Cooking from Around the Sea

JODY NOEL CAMERON

BENEVA PUBLISHING
Brea, California

Publisher's Cataloging-in-Publication Data

Names: Cameron, Jody Noel, 1978- author.
Title: Homestyle Mediterranean : rustic cooking from around the sea / Jody Noel Cameron.
Description: Brea, CA : Beneva Publishing, 2022. | Includes index.
Identifiers: LCCN 2022949664 (print) | ISBN 978-0-9966261-3-2 (paperback) | ISBN 978-0-9966261-7-0 (hardcover) | ISBN 978-0-9966261-4-9 (ebook)
Subjects: LCSH: Cooking, Mediterranean. | Diet--Mediterranean Region. | Cookbooks. | Illustrated works. | BISAC: COOKING / Regional & Ethnic / Mediterranean.
Classification: LCC TX725.M35 C36 2022 (print) | LCC TX725.M35 (ebook) | DDC 641.59/1822--dc23.

ISBN 978-0-9966261-5-6 (LARGE PRINT EDITION)

Library of Congress Control Number: 2022949664
LC record available at https://lccn.loc.gov/2022949664

Copyright © 2022 by Jody Noel Cameron

All rights reserved. No portion of this book may be reproduced in any form without written permission from the publisher or author, except as permitted by U.S. copyright law.

CONTENTS

Introduction	1
Beverages	6
Breakfast	13
Dips & Condiments	44
Appetizers	73
Salads	89
Soups	117
Sides	143
Mains	161
Index	190

"Except the vine,
there is no plant which bears a fruit
of as great importance as the olive."

—Pliny (CE 23-79)

INTRODUCTION

The Mediterranean Diet is considered one of the best diets for overall health. The guidelines are simple and nothing is forbidden. It encourages balance, moderation, and nourishing your body with a rainbow of whole foods. This healthy path may improve your mood, lower your risk of disease, and extend your life. Over time it can lead to gradual, but sustainable weight loss too.

The modern concept was inspired by Mediterranean dietary patterns observed in the 50s and 60s. But the cuisine has been evolving for thousands of years. Early home cooks didn't have access to many ingredients. One of the most nutrient-dense was the olive. Olive trees thrived where other crops wouldn't grow.

Diet is one way to improve your well-being. But it's important to manage stress and to be physically active too. Restorative rituals are also commonplace around the coast, like siesta (Spain), riposo (Italy), and fjaka (Croatia), to name a few. So enjoy a midday cat-nap, or just pause to appreciate the beauty of the world around you.

The Mediterranean includes over 20 countries along the coastlines of Africa, Asia, and Europe. And it's dotted with thousands of islands like Malta, Santorini, and Hvar—Each with a distinct cuisine that has been shaped by local flavors. Let the region be your endless source of inspiration for everyday healthy cooking.

WHAT TO EAT

Nourish your body with minimally processed REAL FOOD!

Eat an abundance of ripe, seasonal **FRUIT & VEGETABLES**. Dried fruit, like apricots, figs, dates, and raisins, are loaded with nutrients too.

LEGUMES—like lentils, beans, and peas, are an excellent source of plant-based protein. Low-sodium canned beans are handy for quick meals.

WHOLE GRAINS—Brown rice, barley, bulgur, farro, millet, and oats. Quinoa and wild rice are pseudo-grain superfoods and they're gluten free.

NUTS & SEEDS—Almonds, walnuts, pistachios, sunflower seeds, pine nuts, pumpkin seeds, etc.

FRESH HERBS & SPICES—Explore spices and go overboard with fresh herbs.

OLIVES & EXTRA-VIRGIN OLIVE OIL—Replace butter, margarine, and other refined oils with extra-virgin olive oil.

EAT MODERATELY

FISH & SEAFOOD—salmon, canned light tuna, cod, mackerel, anchovies, sardines, shrimp, mussels, etc. Enjoy a variety of seafood that's low in mercury and high in omega-3 fatty acids.

POULTRY & EGGS are convenient sources of quality lean protein.

DAIRY—unsweetened yogurt, ricotta, goat cheese, feta cheese, Parmigiano-Reggiano, manchego, blue cheese, etc. Just a pinch of stronger tasting cheese goes a long way to boost flavor.

RED WINE—It's fine to enjoy a glass of red wine with a meal. But you don't have to drink wine to benefit from this lifestyle.

LIMIT OR AVOID

- Limit your intake of red meat. Choose lean cuts and use it to enhance the flavor and texture of a healthy meal.
Meat is used sparingly in Mediterranean cooking.
- Processed meat and cheese, like hot dogs, sausages, and lunch meat.
- Butter, margarine, and refined oils. (Replace with extra-virgin olive oil)
- Refined grains and sugars
- Heavily processed foods

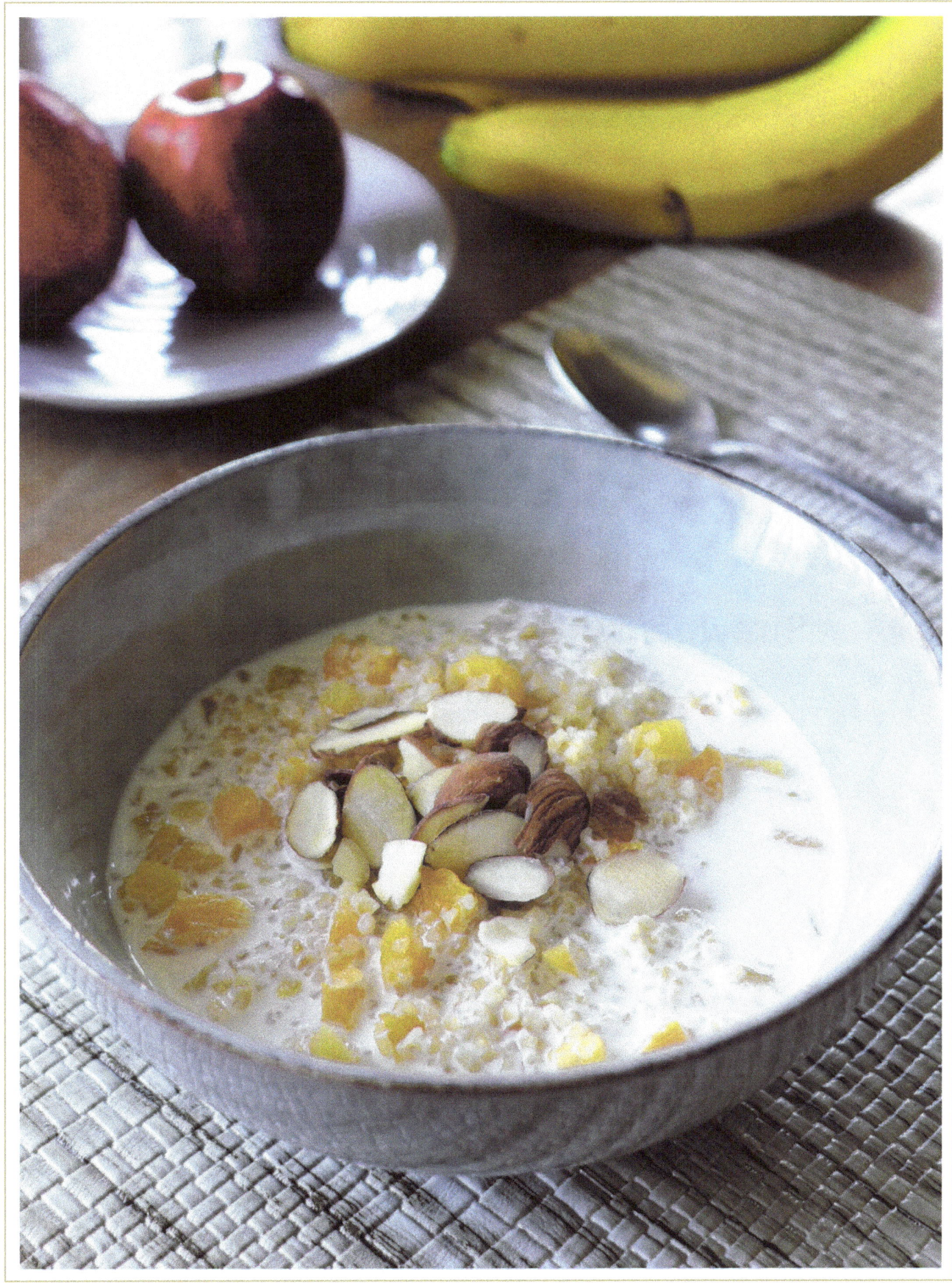

Beverages

Hibiscus Iced Tea

Strawberry Watermelon Quencher

Salted Yogurt Drink

Ginger Milk

Spanish Honey Coffee

Hibiscus Iced Tea

Egyptian pharaohs loved Hibiscus Tea. It's tart like cranberries and may help lower blood pressure. This recipe makes one pitcher of antioxidant-rich hibiscus tea.

2 quarts (8 cups) water, divided
½ cup dried hibiscus (food grade)
1 cinnamon stick
honey or preferred sweetener
fresh lime juice, to taste (optional)
ice (to serve)

1. Simmer five cups of water, hibiscus, and cinnamon stick for 10 minutes. Strain into a pitcher. Sweeten to taste.
2. Add remaining three cups of water.
3. Add lime juice. Chill and serve over ice.

FOR ONE SERVING: pour 1 cup boiling water over 1 tsp. loose hibiscus flowers or one teabag. Add honey, lime, and ground cinnamon if desired. Strain if needed. Chill or serve hot in the colder months.

Strawberry Watermelon Quencher

Watermelons need time to sweeten on the vine. Choose one with a large creamy-yellow patch where it's been sitting in the field.

6-8 cups chopped seedless watermelon
1 cup chopped strawberries, hulled (very ripe)
a squeeze of fresh lemon or lime
ice (to serve)
cold water or sparkling water (optional)
<u>Variation</u>: add some peeled cucumber or fresh mint to the blend.

    1. Liquefy the watermelon and strawberries in a blender. Pour through a fine mesh strainer into a pitcher. Add lemon or lime to taste.
    2. Chill and serve over ice. Or splash some into drinking water or sparkling water for hint of fruit essence.

Salted Yogurt Drink

This refreshing probiotic drink has been a source or nutrients, electrolytes, and hydration for centuries along the eastern Mediterranean. Try it with savory filo-based pastries, kebabs, and grilled foods.

1½ cup plain yogurt
1 cup water
1 tsp. dried mint or a few fresh mint leaves (optional)
pinch sea salt
ice (to serve)

    1. Blend the yogurt, water, mint, and sea salt in a blender until frothy. Serve chilled or over ice.

Ginger Milk

¼ cup chopped fresh ginger
1 cinnamon stick
1 cup water
2-3 cups milk (whole, low-fat, plant-based)
honey or preferred sweetener, to taste

Golden Ginger Milk
Add ½ tsp. ground turmeric, plus a few grinds of black pepper.

Cardamom Milk
Toss a few smashed cardamom pods into the pot.

1. Place the ginger, cinnamon stick, and water into a pot (plus additional spices if using). Simmer until reduced by half.
2. Add the milk and simmer gently for a few more minutes. Keep the heat fairly low and stir often. Milk can boil over and scorch your pan.
3. Sweeten to taste and strain before serving. Enjoy warm or chilled.

Spanish Honey Coffee

¼ cup (per serving) prepared espresso or strong coffee
1 cup milk (whole milk works best)
honey, to taste
dash cinnamon, preferably Ceylon (or ground cardamom)
dash nutmeg (optional)

1. Brew your espresso or very strong coffee.
2. <u>Froth the milk</u>: Place the milk into a jar. Cover and shake vigorously until foamy. Remove the lid. Then microwave 30-60 seconds.
3. <u>To assemble</u>: Add honey to each coffee mug. Pour in a quarter cup of espresso or strong coffee. Spoon at least a half cup of frothy milk over the coffee. Sprinkle with cinnamon and nutmeg.

Arabic-style coffee is a quick dairy and sugar-free option. Brew some strong coffee with a few smashed cardamom pods. Or just add a good pinch of ground cardamom to your coffee cup.

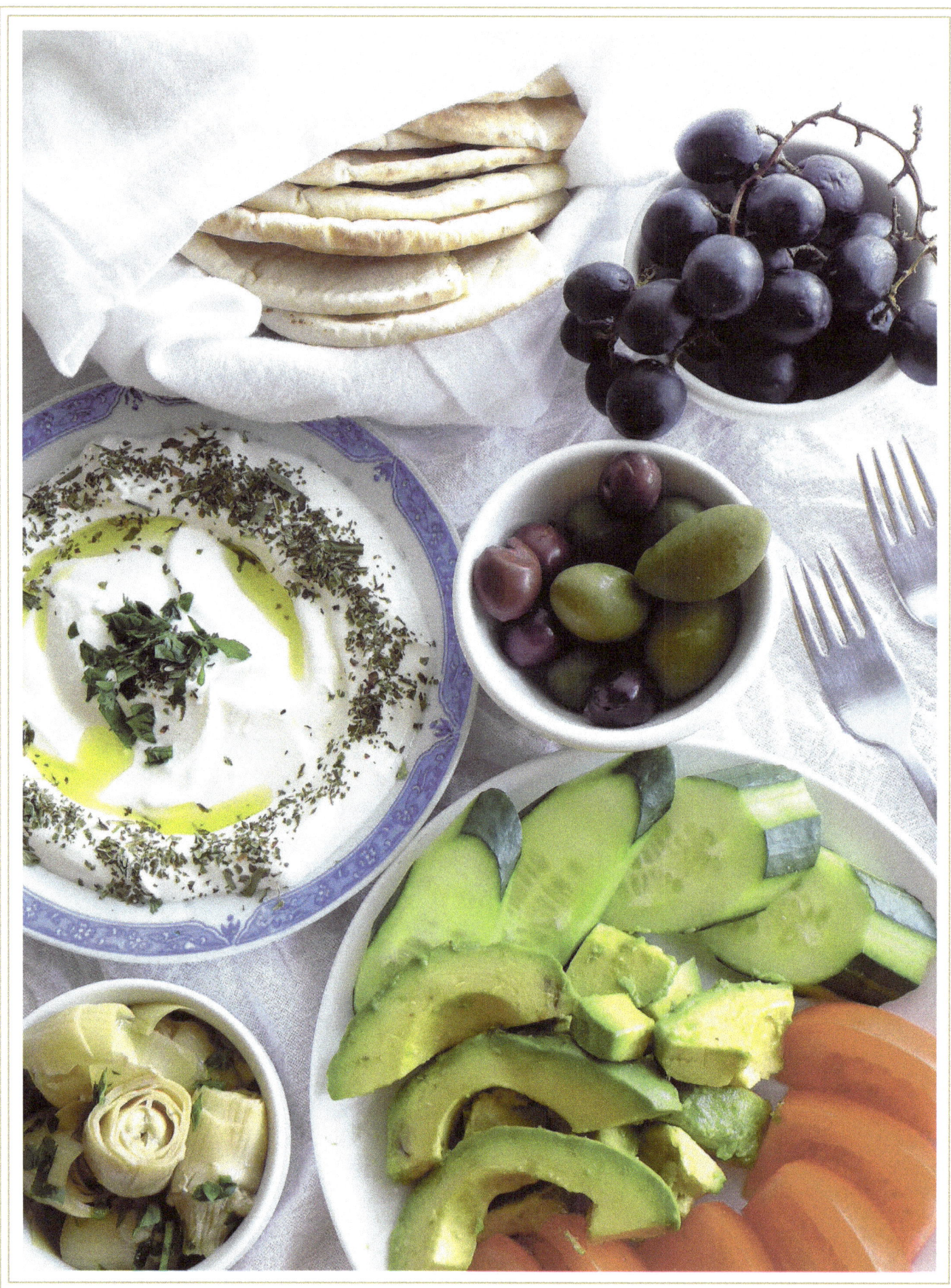

BREAKFAST

Good Morning Graze

Strained Yogurt with Honey & Walnuts

Greek Yogurt with Roasted Strawberries

Labneh Yogurt Spread

Tahini Honey Butter

Catalan Tomato Toast

Olive Oil-Basted Eggs

Tomato Harvest Scramble

Spanish Zucchini Scramble

Istrian Wild Asparagus Fritaja

Balkan Spinach Eggs

Portobello Baked Eggs

Tunisian Protein Bowl with Harissa

Turkish Poached Eggs with Feta-Yogurt Sauce

Quick & Cold Bulgur Cereal

Apricot, Almond & Dark Chocolate Granola Clusters

100% Whole-Wheat Pancakes

with Red Wine Blueberry Compote

Milk & Honey Barley Porridge

Good Morning Graze

Pair your morning coffee with warm conversation and wholesome nibbles. Breakfast is the perfect time to get your graze on!

Which healthy foods would you like to wake up to? Fill an assortment of small bowls and plates with your favorite items—in the style of tapas, mezze, or antipasti. Plate what you can the night before for an easy start.

- Simple salads
- Hard-boiled eggs
- Olives, nuts, and seeds
- Whole grain baked goods
- Fresh fruit (e.g., grapes, berries, sliced melon)
- Dried fruit (e.g., apricots, dates, figs, raisins)
- Healthy dips (e.g., hummus, matbucha, etc.)
- Yogurt and cheese (e.g., feta, labneh, Manchego, etc.)
- Vegetables (e.g., radishes, cucumbers, avocados, tomato wedges)

Strained Yogurt with Honey & Walnuts

Greek-style strained yogurt is a luxurious Mediterranean staple. It's the base of many dips (e.g., tzatziki) and the star of this velvety dish, Yiaourti me Meli. Strained yogurt contains probiotics, calcium, and more protein per serving than unstrained.

Strained Yogurt
1 (32-oz.) container plain whole-milk yogurt

Yiaourti me Meli
honey, to taste
¼ cup chopped walnuts
cinnamon (optional)
fresh fruit (optional)

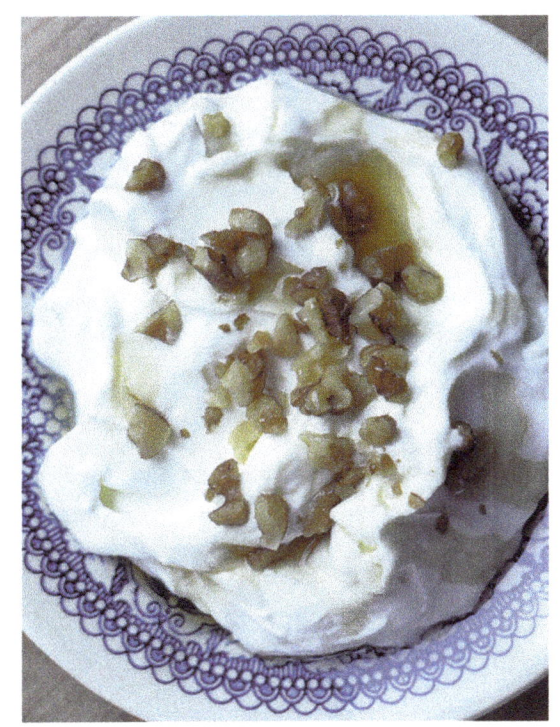

1. Strained Yogurt: Scoop the yogurt into a fine mesh strainer over a bowl. Cover and strain in the refrigerator for 12 to 48 hours. Discard the liquid (whey) as it accumulates. Use as desired.

2. Yiaourti me Meli: Scoop about ¾ cup of the strained yogurt into a bowl. Drizzle with honey. Sprinkle with walnuts and cinnamon. Serve with fresh fruit if desired.

Greek Yogurt with Roasted Strawberries

Spoon these scrumptious strawberries onto yogurt, oatmeal, or whole-wheat pancakes.

1 lb. strawberries
1 Tbsp. honey
1 Tbsp. balsamic vinegar
pinch sea salt
¾ cup (per serving) plain Greek/strained whole-milk, low-fat, or plant-based yogurt

1. Preheat your oven to 350°F. Remove the stems to hull the strawberries. Cut the berries in half. Quarter larger ones.
2. Pile berries onto a parchment-lined baking sheet. Add honey, balsamic, and a pinch of salt. Mix well.
3. Roast for 30 minutes. Set aside to cool. Scrape the berries and juices into a resealable container with a rubber spatula. Refrigerate until ready to use.

Labneh Yogurt Spread

This versatile yogurt cheese is easy to make at home. It's a better spread for your bagel and can thicken soups and sauces without using butter, heavy cream, cornstarch, or flour.

1 (32-oz.) container plain whole-milk yogurt (low-fat dairy is not ideal)
½ tsp. sea salt
accompaniment: flatbread (optional)

1. To make labneh combine the yogurt and salt. Scoop it into a fine mesh strainer over a bowl. Cover and strain in the refrigerator for 48 to 72 hours. Discard the liquid (whey) as it accumulates. The labneh is now ready to use as desired.
2. Spread labneh onto a plate. Sprinkle with fresh or dried herbs (like chives, basil, oregano, thyme, or mint). Drizzle with good extra-virgin olive oil. Serve with warm flatbread.
3. Warm flatbread in an oven preheated to 325°F for 5-10 minutes; microwave for a few seconds; or use a toaster for slightly crisp flatbread halves in seconds.

Tahini Honey Butter

Move over peanut butter. Tahinomelo is delicious on toast, in yogurt, and dipped with fruit. This sweet and nutty duo is found in Macedonia, Cyprus, Greece, and Turkey.

¼ cup tahini sesame paste
¼ cup honey
dash of cinnamon

1. Whisk together equal amounts of tahini and honey. Stir in cinnamon. Adjust the ratio to suit your taste. Refrigerate in an airtight container. Stir before serving.

"Slowly, slowly the sour grape becomes honey."

—Greek proverb

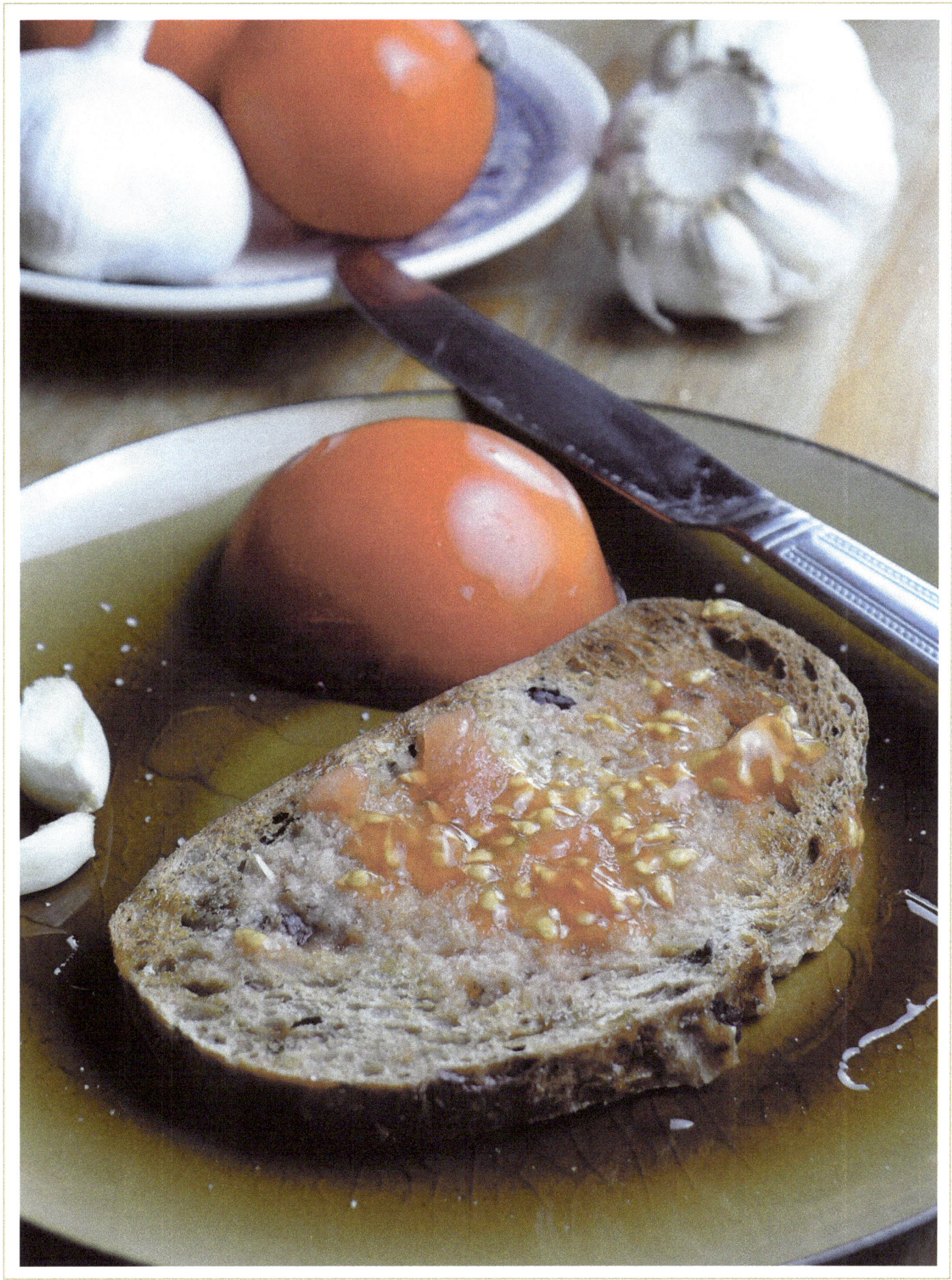

Catalan Tomato Toast

This home style dish is iconic of Catalan cuisine – where frugal farmers would soften stale bread with tomatoes.

1-2 ripe juicy tomatoes, halved
toasted bread
1 garlic clove, halved
sea salt, to taste
good extra-virgin olive oil

Traditional Toppings
olive oil-basted egg, anchovies, thinly sliced Manchego cheese and/or ham (esp., Iberian or Serrano)

1. Grate the open end of each tomato half into a bowl. Discard the skin. (Alternatively, rub the tomato directly onto the bread after the garlic in step 2.)
2. Toast the bread and rub with garlic to leave its essence. Spread tomato onto each piece of toast. Sprinkle with sea salt, then drizzle with extra-virgin olive oil. Enjoy this simple dish as is, or add your choice of topping(s).

Olive Oil-Basted Eggs

Goodbye margarine, butter, and bacon grease. Baste your eggs in olive oil until their edges are golden and crisp.

3 Tbsp. extra-virgin olive oil
2 eggs
sea salt and black pepper, to taste

1. Heat the oil in a non-stick skillet over medium heat. Crack the eggs into the oil.
2. Carefully tilt the pan so that olive oil pools on one side. Repeatedly baste the eggs with a spoon until the edges are browned and crispy and the whites are done to your liking. Remove with a slotted spoon.

Tomato Harvest Scramble

Here's an easy way to use a bumper crop of tomatoes or that one going soft in the fridge.

2 Tbsp. extra-virgin olive oil
2-4 very ripe tomatoes, chopped (or a 14.5 oz. can diced tomatoes)
sea salt and freshly ground black pepper
4 eggs, lightly whisked
¼ cup feta cheese, or more to taste

    1. Warm the oil in a non-stick pan over medium heat. Stir in the tomatoes and season with salt and pepper. Cook until most of the juice has evaporated.
    2. Pour in the eggs and stir occasionally. Cook until the eggs have set. Turn off the heat and sprinkle with feta cheese.

Spanish Zucchini Scramble

Zarangollo is a traditional dish from the Murcian coast.

2 Tbsp. extra-virgin olive oil
½ cup diced onion
1 medium zucchini, diced
sea salt
freshly ground black pepper
½ tsp. dried oregano or thyme (optional)
4 eggs, lightly whisked

1. Heat the oil in a large non-stick pan over medium-high. Sauté the onions and zucchini until tender. Season to taste with salt and pepper. Stir in the herbs if using.
2. Reduce the heat to medium. Pour in the eggs. Stir occasionally and cook for a few minutes, until the eggs have set.

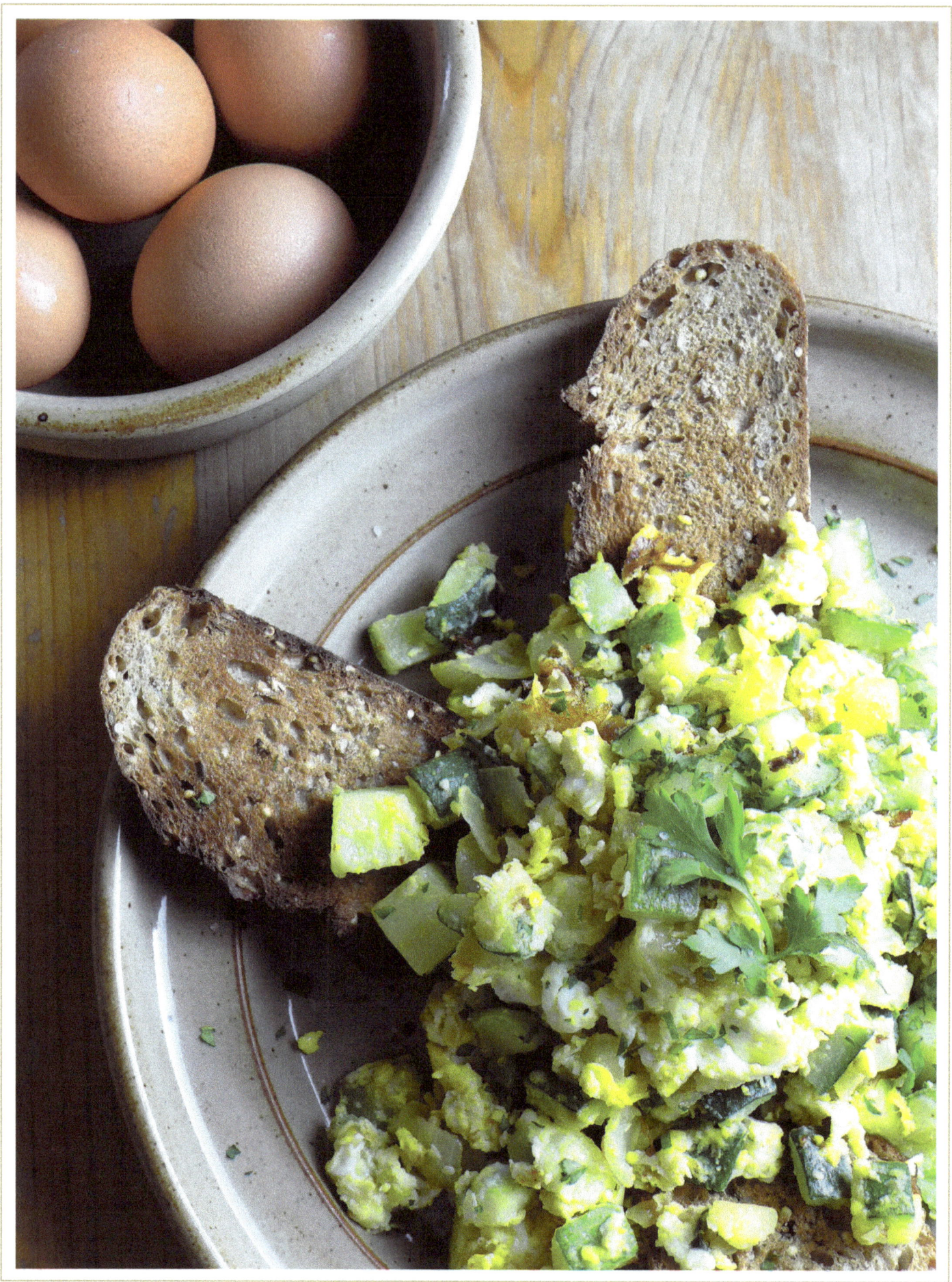

Istrian Wild Asparagus Fritaja

Wild asparagus marks the beginning of springtime in Istria. The annual hunt provides fun, fresh air, and fritaja. Add shaved truffles, prosciutto, fresh herbs, or goat cheese.

1 bunch tender, thin asparagus
2 Tbsp. extra-virgin olive oil
3 scallions, sliced
   (or dice 1 small onion)
fine sea salt
4 eggs, lightly whisked
freshly ground black pepper
aged goat cheese (optional)

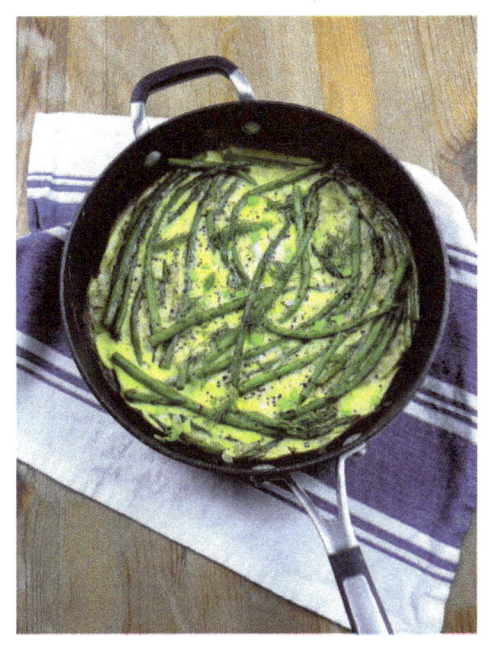

1. Wash asparagus and trim tough ends. Cut into bite-size pieces or leave whole if thin. Heat olive oil in a non-stick pan. Sauté scallions and asparagus with a dash of sea salt until tender (add prosciutto now if using).

2. Add the eggs. Stir occasionally to scramble until eggs are cooked to your liking. Sometimes fritaja is made more like an omelet or frittata. Instead of scrambling, cover the pan for a few minutes to steam the top. Season. Grate cheese over your fritaja for an authentic touch.

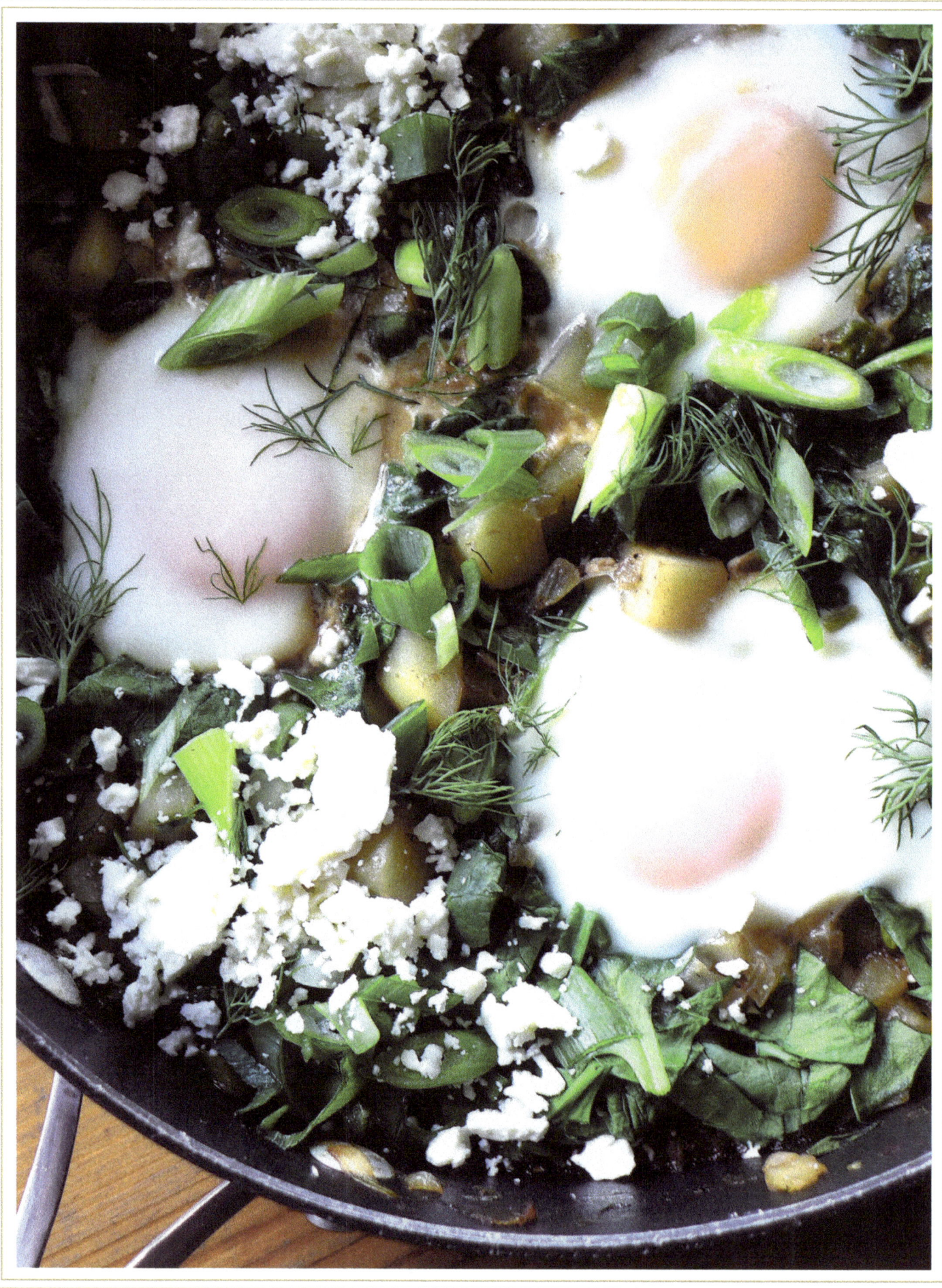

Balkan Spinach Eggs

1½ cups diced potatoes, 1 can white beans, or 1 cup cooked rice (optional)
1 Tbsp. extra-virgin olive oil
4 scallions, sliced (or 1 small onion, diced; One scallion is all growth from the root.)
2 garlic cloves, minced
sea salt and black pepper, to taste
pinch nutmeg
¼ cup water
4 handfuls fresh spinach or any baby greens (**use up your greens here!**)
2-4 eggs
feta cheese
accompaniment: crusty bread

    1. Optionally add potatoes, beans, or rice for a heartier breakfast — **any leftovers?** First boil your potatoes in salted water until fork tender; drain. Alternatively, drain and rinse a can of beans. For a more traditional version, measure out a cup of cooked rice instead. Set aside.

    2. Heat olive oil in a wide pan over medium heat. Cook scallions and garlic for a few minutes to infuse the oil with flavor.

3. Stir in the potatoes, beans, or rice if using.

4. Season with sea salt, black pepper, and nutmeg. Add the water and shake the pan to distribute. Pile on the spinach.

5. Once the spinach has wilted, make a few indentations in the mixture. Then crack an egg into each. Cover. Cook for about 3 minutes, or until the eggs have set to your liking. Crumble with feta and serve with crusty bread.

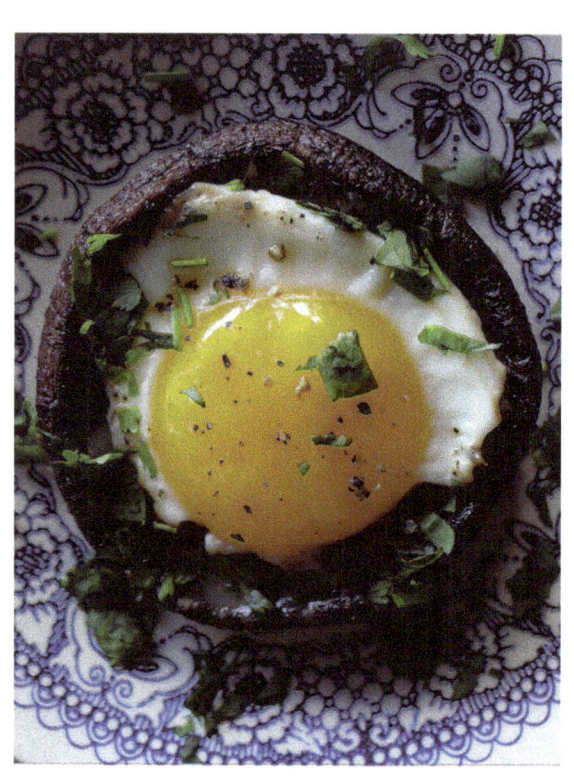

Portobello Baked Eggs

2 portobello mushroom caps
extra-virgin olive oil
sea salt
freshly ground black pepper
2 eggs
chopped parsley or chives (to garnish)

1. Prep the mushrooms: Preheat your oven to 425°F and line a sheet pan with parchment. Wipe mushrooms clean with a damp paper towel. Carefully scrape out the gills with the tip of a spoon to create a bowl. Rub with a thin coating of oil and season with salt and pepper. Bake upright on the pan for 15 minutes.
2. Remove from the oven and drain excess liquid. Crack an egg into each cap. Season the eggs. Bake for 10 minutes or until the whites have set to your liking. Sprinkle with chopped parsley or chives.

*To dress up this easy breakfast add some pesto, marinara, baby spinach, or cheese (e.g., Gruyère, Swiss cheese, goat cheese, parmesan) into the mushroom before adding the eggs.

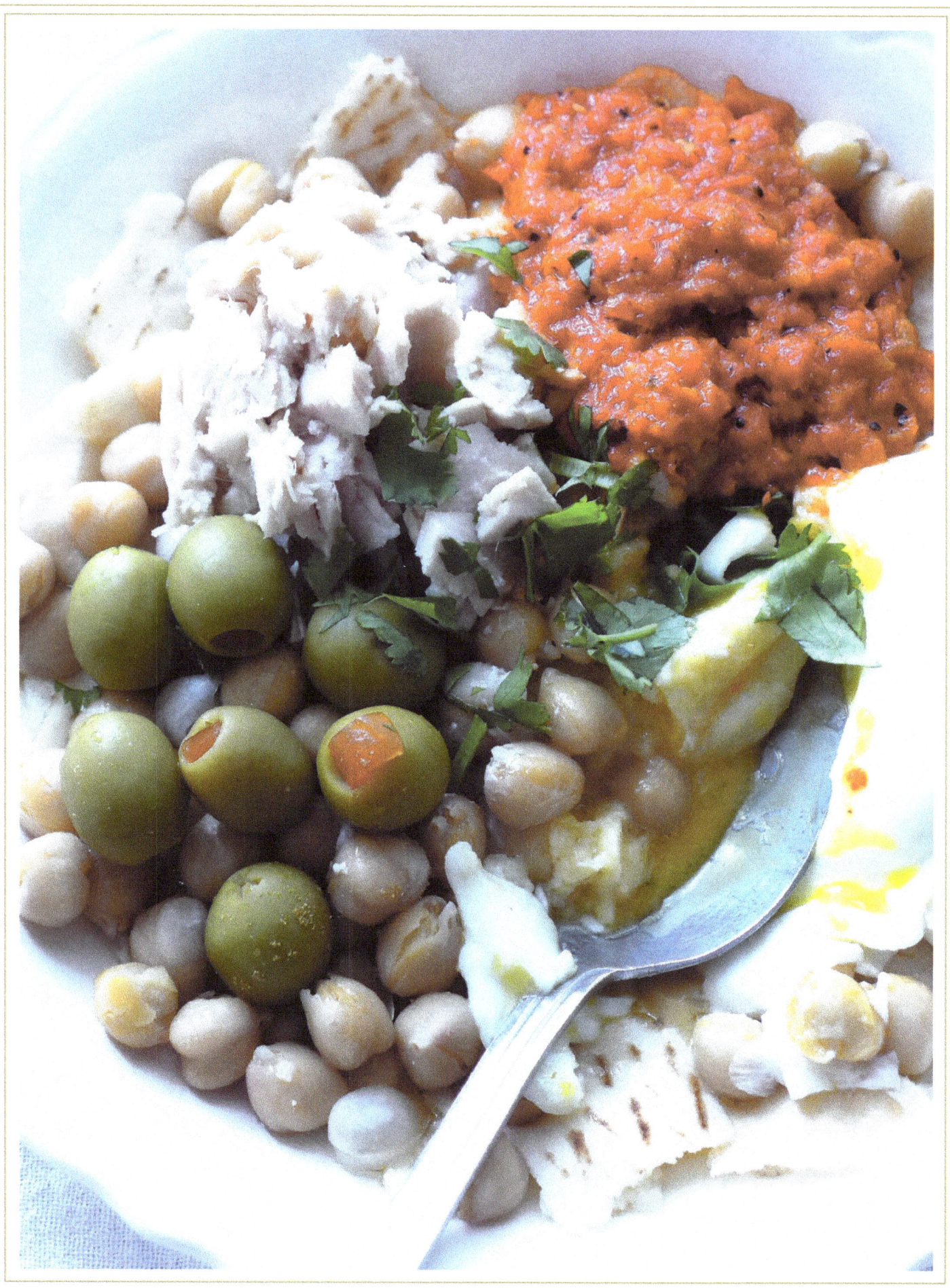

Tunisian Protein Bowl with Harissa

Mediterranean cooking is frugal. Especially when it comes to stale bread, which is repurposed in soups, salads, and casseroles.

This everday Tunisian breakfast begins with hot, cumin-scented chickpea soup that's ladled over bits of bread. But the toppings—poached eggs, tuna, capers, olives, and fiery harissa are why you'll fall in love with lablabi.

Chickpea Soup
2 Tbsp. extra-virgin olive oil
1 Tbsp. minced garlic
1 tsp. ground cumin
2 (15-oz.) canned chickpeas, drained and rinsed
1 quart (4 cups) low-sodium vegetable or chicken stock
water (to cover)

stale flat bread or rustic loaf, torn into bits
1 egg (per serving)
capers and/or olives
1 (5-oz.) can tuna, drained
1 lemon, halved
harissa or other hot sauce

1. <u>Chickpea Soup</u>: Heat the oil in a pot and cook garlic and cumin for about a minute. Stir in chickpeas and stock. Cover with water by two inches. Simmer for 30 minutes. Smash a third of the chickpeas with your spoon.

2. Poach the eggs 2-3 minutes in gently bubbling water (optionally with a splash of vinegar). Or poach the eggs directly in the soup broth.

3. <u>Assembly</u>: Place a handful of torn bread into each bowl. Ladle some chickpeas and broth onto the bread to soften it. Top with poached egg. Sprinkle with more cumin. Scatter capers, olives, and bits of tuna. Finish with a squeeze of lemon and a spoonful of harissa. Enjoy!

<u>Harissa</u>
2.5 oz. California, Ancho, or other mild chilis
2 Tbsp. extra-virgin olive oil
2 Tbsp. lemon juice
2 garlic cloves, peeled
¾ tsp. sea salt, or more to taste
½ cup fresh water
1 tsp. paprika
½ tsp. cayenne pepper, or to taste
½ tsp. ground cumin
½ tsp. ground caraway or coriander

1. Crack off the dried chili stems and shake out the seeds. Break into smaller pieces. Toast the chilis in a large pan. Transfer to a bowl and cover with boiling water. Soak for 30 minutes.

2. Drain and transfer to a food processor. Add the oil, lemon, garlic, salt, and fresh water.

3. Briefly toast the spices in the same pan until fragrant. Add them to the mixture and blend until smooth. Optionally press through a fine mesh strainer with a rubber spatula. Refrigerate in an airtight container. Your harissa will last longer if covered by a thin layer of olive oil.

Turkish Poached Eggs with Feta-Yogurt Sauce

Ottoman sultans enjoyed Çılbır in the 15th century. A bit of feta cheese (a Bulgarian twist) gives this version big flavor.

Chili Oil
¼ cup extra-virgin olive oil
2 tsp. Aleppo pepper or paprika
pinch sea salt

Feta-Yogurt Sauce
1 small garlic clove
pinch sea salt
¼ cup feta cheese (optional)
1½ cup (room temperature) plain yogurt
sea salt and black pepper, to taste

1-2 poached eggs (per serving)
accompaniment: warm flat bread

    1. <u>Chili Oil</u>: Warm oil in a pot over medium heat. Swirl in the red pepper and salt. Remove from heat and set aside.
    2. <u>Feta-Yogurt Sauce</u>: Finely mince the garlic with a pinch of sea salt. Smash it into a paste using the flat side of your knife. Place the garlic into a bowl. Add the feta cheese and smash it with a fork. Add the yogurt, salt, and pepper. Mix well.
    3. Poach the eggs for two to three minutes in gently simmering water (optionally add a splash of vinegar to the water). Remove with a slotted spatula and drain on sturdy paper towel.
    4. Divide the yogurt sauce among two plates. Top with the eggs and drizzle with chili oil. Serve with bread.

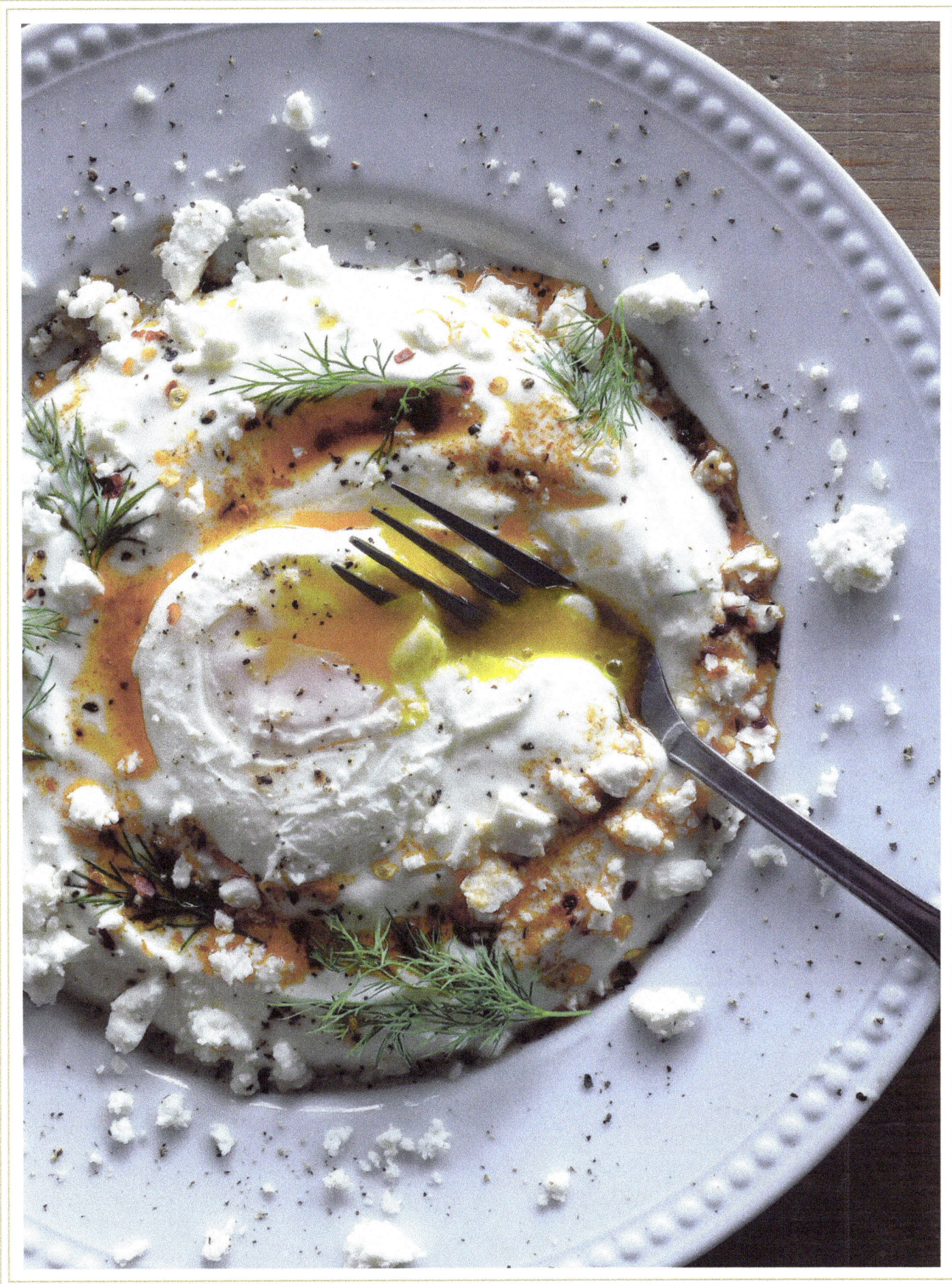

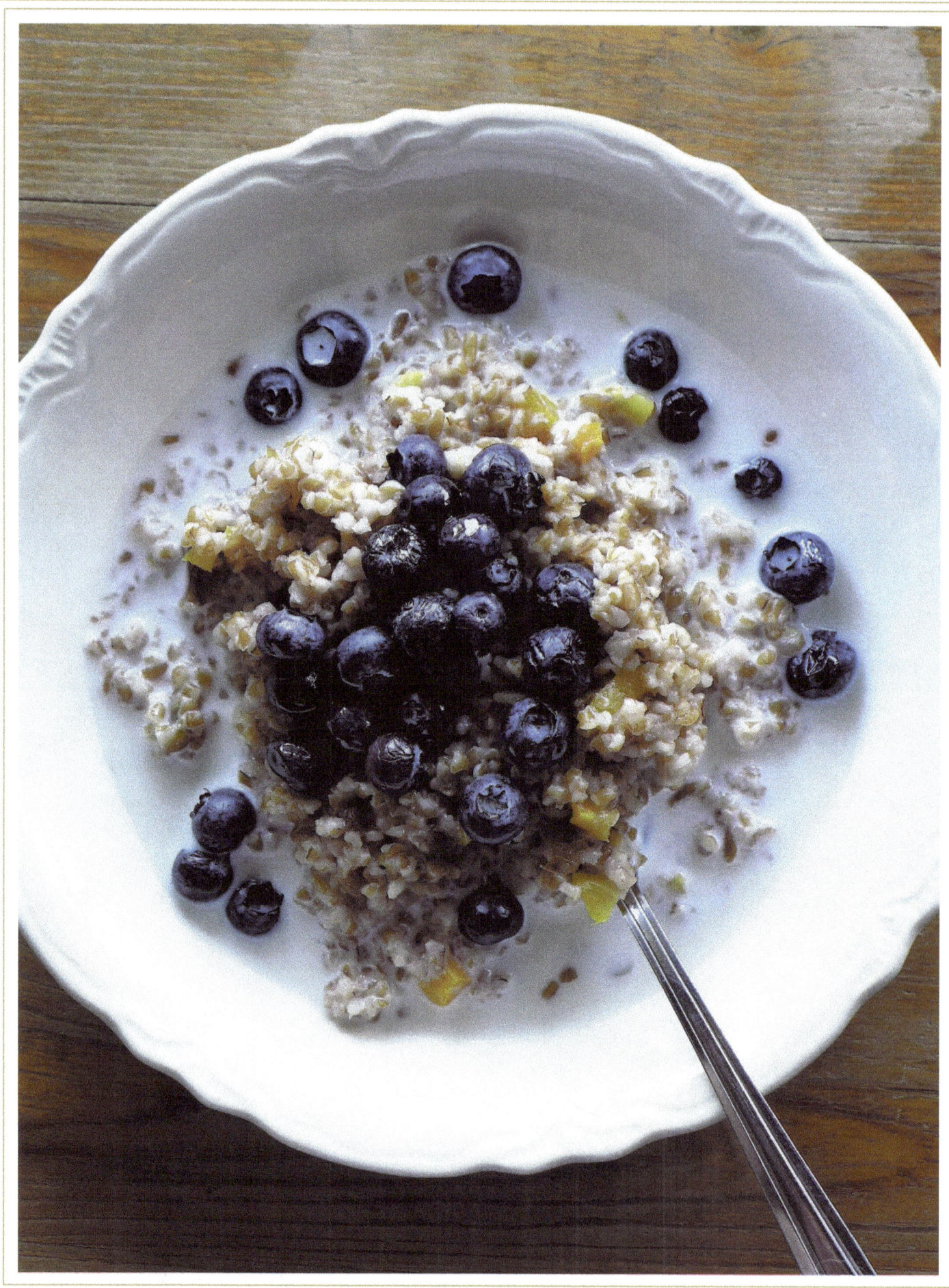

Quick & Cold Bulgur Cereal

This Eastern staple only requires a quick soak before using. Fine bulgur cereal may be the easiest way to consume more whole grains.

¼ cup fine bulgur wheat (#1) (contains gluten)
1-2 Tbsp. dried fruit, like raisins, cherries, chopped apricot
pinch of sea salt
½ cup boiling hot water
milk of your choice
honey or preferred sweetener, to taste (optional)

1. Combine the bulgur, dried fruit, salt, and hot water in a bowl. Cover and set aside for 15 minutes. The bulgur and dried fruit (if using) will rehydrate and absorb most of the water. Drain excess water and fluff with a fork.
2. Serve with cold milk and sweeten as desired. Top with nuts, berries, bananas, cocoa nibs, coconut, etc.

*Medium and coarse ground bulgur must be boiled first. Simmer 1 cup bulgur with 2 cups water; covered; for 12 minutes. Off heat, let rest for another 10 minutes before serving. Fluff with a fork.

Apricot, Almond & Dark Chocolate Granola Clusters

½ cup extra-virgin olive oil
½ cup honey (or maple syrup)
1 tsp. pure vanilla extract or paste
1 tsp. cinnamon
½ tsp. ground cardamom
½ tsp. fine sea salt
3 cups old-fashioned oats
½ cup almonds (or any nuts/seeds)
⅓ cup chopped dried apricots (or other dried fruit; or top with fresh berries)
½ cup chopped dark chocolate or chips (>70% cacao)

1. Preheat oven to 300°F and line a sheet pan with parchment. Whisk together the oil, honey, vanilla, cinnamon, cardamom, and salt. Mix in oats and almonds.
2. Scoop mixture onto pan. Firmly press the mound into a compact rectangle about ½-inch in height. This method should result in chunky oat clusters! Bake for 20 minutes.
3. Break the rectangle into large chunks with a spatula. Rotate the pan and bake for another 10 minutes or until lightly golden.

4. Set the pan aside for about an hour to cool. The granola will crisp-up as it sits. Toss in the apricots and chocolate when completely cool.

5. Store in an airtight container at room temperature. Enjoy this high-energy food with cold milk, on yogurt, or as a portable snack.

100% Whole-Wheat Pancakes with Red Wine Blueberry Compote

Pancakes may not seem Mediterranean. But in ancient Greek theaters, they were sold from concession stands at intermission.

1 cup milk
2 tsp. vinegar
1 egg
1 Tbsp. extra-virgin olive oil (plus more for the pan)
1 Tbsp. honey (or pure maple syrup)
1 tsp. pure vanilla extract
1 cup whole-wheat flour
½ tsp. baking powder
½ tsp. baking soda
¼ tsp. fine sea salt

1. Combine the milk and vinegar in a small bowl. Set aside for five minutes. In a larger bowl, whisk the rest of the wet ingredients: egg, oil, honey, and vanilla. Stir in the milk mixture too.

2. Combine the dry ingredients, then add them to the wet mixture. Stir to combine, but don't overmix. It's fine to leave a few lumps. (fold in some blueberries at this point for blueberry pancakes.)

3. Heat a large lightly-oiled skillet over medium. When hot, pour about a third of a cup of batter for each pancake. When bubbles rise to the top and the bottom is lightly browned, flip and cook for another minute or so. Repeat to use the remaining batter.

> A tavola non s'invecchia.
> "One does not grow old at the table."
>
> —Italian expression

Red Wine Blueberry Compote

½ cup red wine
2 Tbsp. honey
½ tsp. lemon zest
¼ tsp. cinnamon
pinch sea salt
2 cups fresh or frozen blueberries
1 tsp. lemon juice

1. Place ingredients (except lemon juice) into a medium non-reactive pot. Simmer over medium heat until the wine has reduced and the fruit has broken down to form a chunky sauce. Remove from heat and stir in the lemon juice. The sauce will thicken as it cools – thin with water as needed.

For a smooth pourable sauce
Process in a blender or food processor until smooth. Press through a fine mesh strainer with a rubber spatula. Refrigerate if not using right away.

Milk & Honey Barley Porridge

The plant-based diet of elite Roman gladiators was mostly beans and barley. Barley provides more fiber than oats. Even pearled barley is rich in beta glucan, a soluble fiber known for its ability to lower cholesterol.

½ cup pearled barley, rinsed (contains gluten)
2 cups water
1 cup milk of your choice (plus more to serve)
1 Tbsp. honey (or sweetener of your choice)
¼ tsp. sea salt
1 tsp. pure vanilla extract (optional)

1. Bring the barley, water, milk, honey, and sea salt to a boil. Reduce the heat to low, cover, and gently simmer until tender, about 40 minutes. Stir occasionally.
2. Stir in the vanilla. Add more milk and honey as desired.

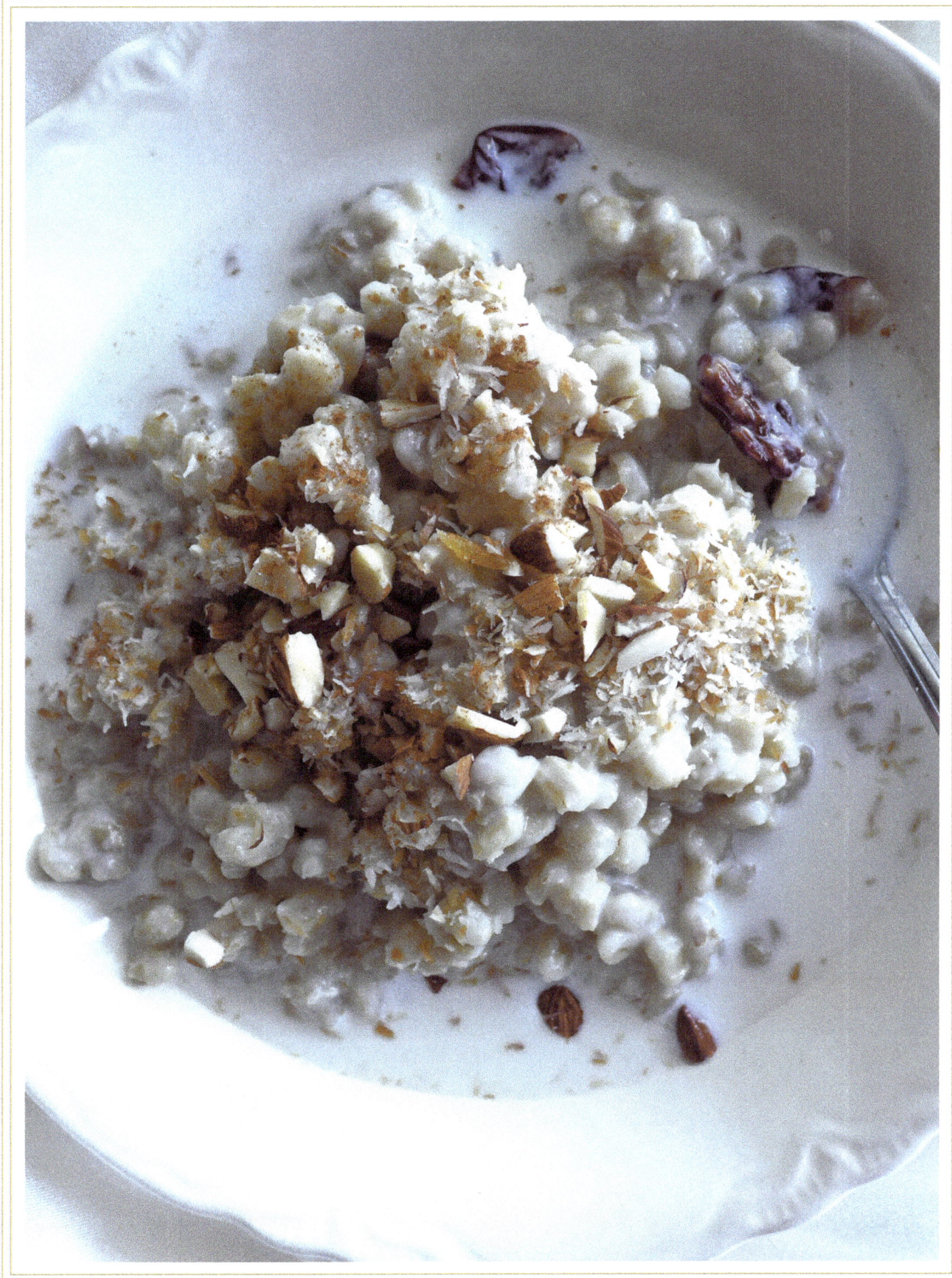

DIPS & CONDIMENTS

Crostini Bites

Garlic Bruschetta Toast

Baked Pita Chips

Tuscan Dipping Oil

Basil Pomodoro

Greek Salsa

Zhoug Hot Sauce

Olive Spread

Onion Marmalade

Mandarin Fig Jam

Cucumber Tzatziki

Spicy Whipped Feta Dip

Eggplant Mutabal

Roasted Jalapeno Carrot Dip

Tomato Matbucha

Santorini Yellow Pea Dip

Mujadara Lentil Dip

Classic Hummus
Red Pepper Hummus
Black Olive Hummus
Pickled Beet Hummus
Jalapeno Hummus
Roasted Garlic Hummus

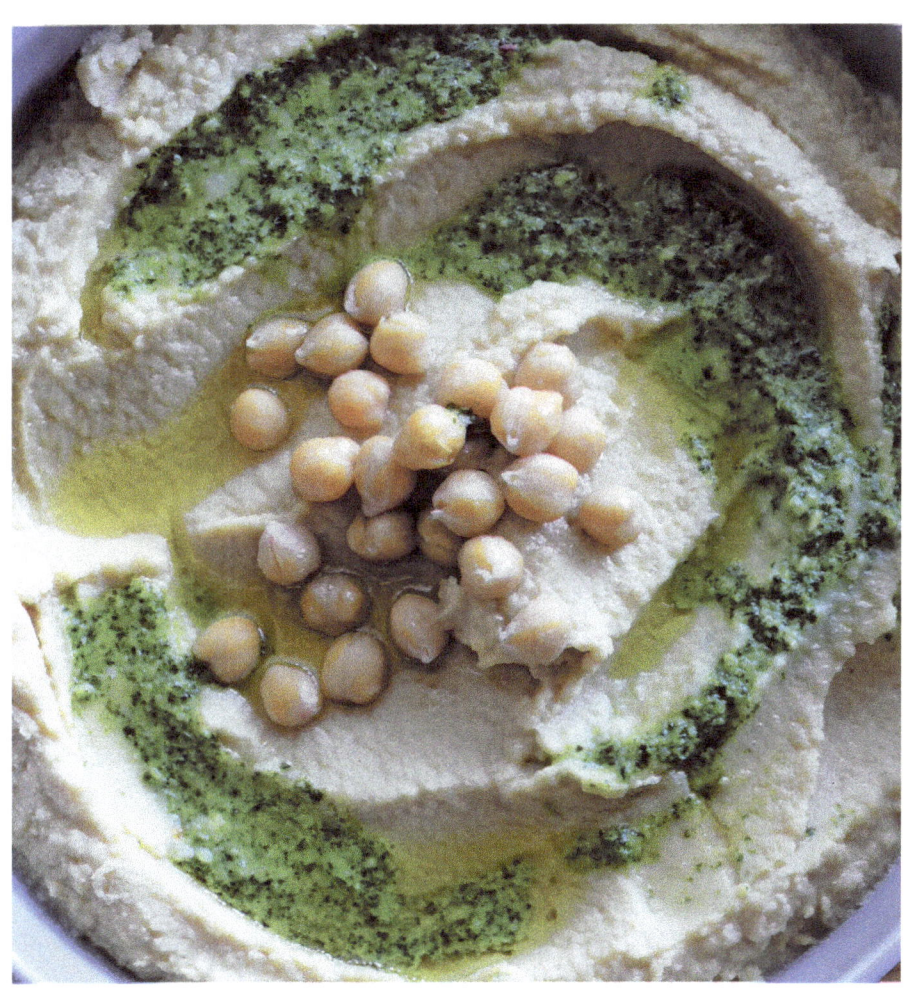

Crostini Bites

Crostini, "little crusts" in Italian, are the perfect foundation for bite-sized appetizers. Crostini can be baked in advance. Store in an airtight container or bag to keep it dry and crisp. Add toppings just before serving.

1 baguette or ficelle, which is a thinner loaf (fresh or stale)
extra-virgin olive oil
fine sea salt

1. Preheat oven to 350°F. Line a baking sheet with parchment paper. Diagonally cut ½-inch thick pieces with a serrated knife.
2. Brush both sides with olive oil and space apart on the baking sheet. Hold your fingers about a foot above the bread and lightly sprinkle a pinch or two of sea salt. Bake until crisp, about 12 to 15 minutes.

Garlic Bruschetta Toast

Modern garlic bread descends from bruschetta. But this bread is simply rubbed with garlic and splashed with good extra-virgin olive oil. Garlicky chopped tomatoes, cannellini beans, and boiled Tuscan kale are just a few traditional toppings.

1-2 slices from a rustic bread loaf, fresh or stale (per person)
1 garlic clove, cut in half
extra-virgin olive oil
fine sea salt

1. Prepare just before serving. Cut loaf into ½-inch slices with a serrated knife.
2. Toast with a toaster, grill, or oven preheated to 425°F. Bake for about 4 minutes on each side.
3. Remove from the oven and rub with a freshly cut end of garlic. Drizzle with extra-virgin olive oil. Sprinkle with sea salt and top as desired.

Baked Pita Chips

4 pita rounds (fresh or stale)
extra-virgin olive oil
fine sea salt

Seasoning Ideas

- Spices: pepper, garlic powder, sumac, cumin, or cayenne
- Herbs: oregano, basil, or thyme
- Blends: Italian, Cajun, Greek - or spinkle with parmesan cheese or citrus zest.

1. Preheat oven to 350°F. Brush a thin layer of olive oil onto whole pitas. Sprinkle with sea salt and your choice of seasonings. Cut into wedges.
2. Space apart on a baking sheet. Bake until crisp and golden, 10-12 minutes. Store in an airtight container or resealable plastic bag.

Tuscan Dipping Oil for Raw Vegetables & Bread

1 tsp. dried oregano
½ tsp. crushed rosemary
½ tsp. garlic powder
½ tsp. sea salt
¼ tsp. freshly ground black pepper
¼ tsp. red pepper flakes
½ cup extra-virgin olive oil
splash balsamic vinegar (optional)
parmesan cheese (optional)

accompaniments:
crusty bread or seasonal vegetables: artichoke hearts, young asparagus, radishes, celery, carrots, tomatoes, green beans, cucumbers, fennel, cauliflower, etc.

1. Combine herbs and spices in a jar and shake well.
2. Pour the olive oil into a shallow dipping bowl. Add some of the spice mix. Splash with balsamic and sprinkle with parmesan if desired.
3. Warm your bread in an oven preheated to 350°F for 5-10 minutes. Or prepare an assortment of raw vegetables.

Basil Pomodoro

Top grilled chicken, fish, or garlicky bruschetta toast – for Bruschetta al Pomodoro, the classic Italian antipasto.

3 Tbsp. extra-virgin olive oil
1 small garlic clove, crushed into a paste with a dash of sea salt
8 fresh basil leaves, chopped
4 large plum tomatoes, seeded and diced
fine sea salt, to taste

1. Combine the ingredients and season well with sea salt. Cover and refrigerate for about an hour before serving.

Greek Salsa

Enjoy with pita chips or as a fresh topping for grilled chicken or salmon.

¼ cup finely diced red onion
¼ cup chopped Kalamata olives
3 Tbsp. extra-virgin olive oil
1 Tbsp. red wine vinegar
1 Tbsp. minced peperoncini
1 Tbsp. chopped parsley leaves
1 tsp. dried oregano
2 Roma tomatoes, seeded and finely diced
1 cup finely diced English cucumber
fine sea salt and black pepper, to taste
½ cup crumbled feta cheese

1. Combine the onions, olives, olive oil, vinegar, peperoncini, parsley, and oregano in a large bowl.
2. Add the tomatoes and cucumbers. Season with salt and pepper. Mix well.
3. Refrigerate for 30 minutes. Gently toss in the feta just before serving.

Zhoug Hot Sauce

Kick up plain hummus with this fiery herbaceous sauce or drizzle it over roasted meat, vegetables, eggs, or rice.

1 large bunch of cilantro, leaves and tender stems
¼ cup extra-virgin olive oil
1 jalapeno, seeds removed
2 garlic cloves, peeled
fresh lemon juice, to taste
½ tsp. ground cumin
½ tsp. ground coriander
¼ tsp. ground cardamom
¼ tsp. red pepper flakes (optional)
sea salt, to taste

1. Process in a blender or food processor. Refrigerate.

Olive Spread

Ancient Romans and Greeks enjoyed olive spread with fresh cheese. They called it <u>Epityrum</u>, which means "over cheese"!

1 cup pitted Kalamata olives
2 tsp. fresh thyme leaves (½ tsp. dried thyme)
1 tsp. lemon juice
1 garlic clove, roughly chopped
freshly ground black pepper, to taste
¼ cup extra-virgin olive oil

1. Blend the ingredients until smooth in a small food processor.

Onion Marmalade

2 Tbsp. extra-virgin olive oil
3 large onions, sliced or diced
½ cup white wine or water
1 Tbsp. balsamic vinegar
1 Tbsp. honey
½ tsp. sea salt, more to taste

1. Heat the oil in a wide sauté pan. Stir in the onions. Cook until golden brown over medium-high heat, about 15 minutes. Stir occasionally.

2. Carefully stir in the wine to deglaze the pan. Add the balsamic, honey, and sea salt. Reduce the heat to medium. Cook until the onions break down, becoming thick and jammy. Stir often and add water as needed.

3. Set aside to cool. Refrigerate and use within a few days. Spread onto sandwiches (awesome addition to grilled cheese), wraps, grilled chicken, burgers, and on crackers with fresh cheese.

Mandarin Fig Jam

Figs are one of the first plants to be cultivated by humans. They're a source of prebiotics, antioxidants, and minerals. Pair this with goat cheese, ricotta, or labneh, on toast or crostini.

½ cup dried figs, chopped (e.g., Mission figs)
½ cup water
4 mandarin oranges, juiced (e.g., clementines; Substitute: ½ cup orange juice)
1 tsp. mandarin orange zest
pinch sea salt
½ lemon

1. Combine ingredients (except for the lemon) in a pot. Simmer until the figs are soft and the liquid has reduced by half, about 10 minutes.
2. Set aside to cool slightly, then squeeze in the lemon juice. Process in a small food processor until smooth and spreadable. The jam will thicken as it cools, so thin with a bit of water if necessary.

Cucumber Tzatziki

1½ cups thick Greek-style yogurt (or strain whole milk plain yogurt overnight to thicken)
½ English seedless cucumber (If using an American Cucumber, first peel the waxy skin and scrape out the seeds.)
sea salt (to draw out moisture)
2 Tbsp. extra-virgin olive oil
1 Tbsp. red wine vinegar
1 Tbsp. chopped dill or spearmint (optional; or add a pinch of dried mint to make Cypriot talatouri.)
1 garlic clove, crushed into a paste
sea salt and freshly ground black pepper, to taste

1. Grate or mince the cucumber. Transfer to a fine mesh strainer and toss generously with sea salt. Set aside for at least 30 minutes. Press or squeeze out as much liquid as you can.
2. Combine the cucumber with the rest of the ingredients. Season to taste with salt and pepper. Cover and chill for at least an hour before serving.

Spicy Whipped Feta Dip

2 roasted red bell peppers
1 cup (4-oz.) brined feta cheese, roughly chopped
½ cup plain Greek-style yogurt
3 Tbsp. extra-virgin olive oil
2 Tbsp. lemon juice
1 tsp. dried oregano
cayenne pepper, to taste

1. Roasted peppers from the jar make this dip quick and easy. But roasting fresh peppers is simple too. Preheat your oven to 425°F. Roast the peppers, turning occasionally, on a sheet pan for 30 minutes or until the skin is partially charred.
2. Immediately transfer to an air-tight container to steam for 15 minutes. Core the peppers and peel off the skin.
3. Pulse the peppers a few times in a food processor. Then add the rest of the ingredients. Add heat with cayenne pepper. Process until smooth, scraping down the sides once or twice. Refrigerate for at least an hour before serving. Scoop with warm flatbread, pita chips, or vegetables.

Eggplant Mutabal

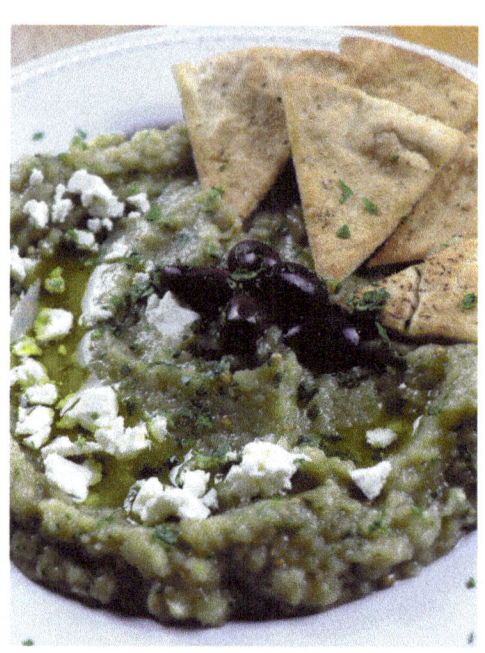

2 eggplants
¼ cup tahini sesame paste
¼ cup Greek-style yogurt (optional)
1 lemon, juiced
2 garlic cloves, crushed into a paste
½ tsp. fine sea salt, or more to taste
extra-virgin olive oil (to drizzle)

1. Preheat oven to 400°F. Pierce eggplants several times with a sharp knife. Roast for 45 minutes on a sheet pan. Set aside to cool completely.
2. Cut the eggplants open and scrape their pulp into a food processor. Add the tahini, yogurt, lemon juice, garlic, and salt. Process until smooth or leave it chunky-style. Or, just smash the ingredients together with a fork.
3. Serve with a splash of good extra-virgin olive oil. Garnish with chopped herbs or pomegranate arils if you wish.

Roasted Jalapeno Carrot Dip

1 lb. (about 8) carrots, peeled and cut into ½-inch pieces
2 jalapenos, cored
1 Tbsp. extra-virgin olive oil
sea salt and black pepper, to taste

2 garlic cloves, peeled
½ tsp. ground cumin
¼ tsp. ground caraway (substitute: coriander)
1 Tbsp. lemon juice
¼ to ½ cup water, to thin

1. Preheat your oven to 425°F and line a sheet pan with parchment. Pile the jalapenos and carrots onto the center of the pan and drizzle with olive oil. Season to taste with salt and pepper. Toss well. Space the pieces apart and roast for 30 minutes or until fork tender.
2. Place the carrots, jalapenos, garlic, spices, and lemon juice into a food processor or blender. Process until smooth, scraping down the sides as needed. Thin with water. Season to taste with more sea salt.
3. Dip with sliced vegetables, crackers, and pita—or use as a side dish with roasted chicken or vegetables.

Tomato Matbucha

Roasted peppers, tomatoes, and garlic simmer low and slow to concentrate this Moroccan Jewish condiment. Sop it up with challah or pita, kick up plain hummus with a fiery scoop, and use it to braise fish (chraime) and eggs (shakshuka).

2 bell peppers, any color
(**Substitute 1 (16-oz.) jar of drained roasted red peppers for Quick Matbucha**)
¼ cup extra-virgin olive oil (plus more to drizzle)
½ cup diced onion
2 jalapenos, minced (or instead add ½ tsp. cayenne when adding the paprika)
1 Tbsp. minced garlic
1 (28-oz.) can diced tomatoes
1 tsp. paprika
½ tsp. smoked paprika
½ tsp. sea salt, or more to taste

1. Roast the peppers (or save time with jarred peppers). Preheat your oven to 425°F. Roast on a sheet pan, turning occasionally, for 30 minutes or until the skin is charred. Immediately transfer to an air-tight container or resealable plastic bag to steam for 15 minutes. Peel off the skin and chop the peppers.

2. Heat the oil in a wide, sturdy pot. Cook the onions, jalapenos, and garlic for a few minutes without browning.

3. Pour in the tomatoes, paprikas, and salt. Gently simmer over low heat until the vegetables break down and the liquid evaporates. Stir occasionally and smash the vegetables as they cook. Serve drizzled with olive oil.

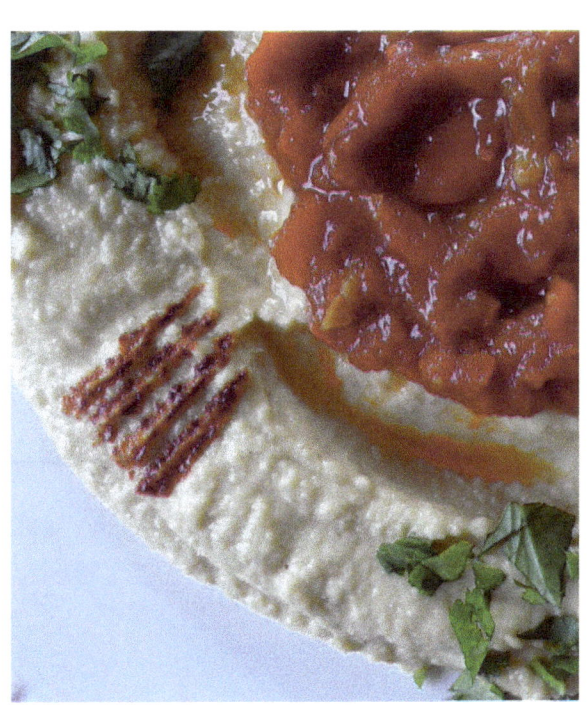

Santorini Yellow Pea Dip

Visit Santorini Island by way of this regional dip made from yellow split peas.

2 Tbsp. extra-virgin olive oil (plus more to drizzle)
1 large red onion, diced (reserve ¼ cup to garnish)
1 Tbsp. minced garlic
2-3 thyme sprigs (or ½ tsp. dried thyme)
1 bay leaf
sea salt
1 cup yellow split peas, inspected for pebbles and rinsed
water, to cover
½ lemon
1 Tbsp. capers, rinsed and patted dry (optional)

    1. Heat the oil in a pot. Add the onions, garlic, thyme, bay leaf, and a dash of salt. Cook until the onions are translucent (without browning the garlic).
    2. Pour the peas into the pot and cover with water. Bring to a boil. Cover and reduce heat to low. Simmer 45 minutes or until the peas a mushy. Stir occasionally and add more water as needed.
    3. Discard thyme sprigs and bay leaf. Squeeze with

lemon and season with sea salt. Purée with an immersion blender or food processor.

    4. Spread the dip into a shallow bowl. Drizzle with extra-virgin olive oil. Garnish with diced onion and capers. Serve with pita or grilled fish as a side.

Mujadara Lentil Dip

Inspired by the Levantine dish, this smooth Mujadara-style dip features caramelized onions and a touch of spice.

3 Tbsp. extra-virgin olive oil
2 onions, diced
sea salt
3½ cups water, divided
3 garlic cloves, minced
1 tsp. ground cumin
¾ tsp. ground coriander
½ tsp. black pepper
¼ tsp. turmeric
1 cup dried lentils, inspected for pebbles and rinsed
1 bay leaf
1 lemon, halved

1. Brown the onions in the oil with a pinch of sea salt over medium heat, stirring occasionally. Once they're rusty brown, deglaze the pan with ½ cup of water. Stir well to loosen the fond stuck to the bottom of the pot. Set aside a third of the onions to use as a topping later.

2. Stir in the rest of the water, garlic, spices, lentils, and bay leaf. Bring to a boil. Then reduce the heat to low. Cover and simmer 25 minutes or until the lentils are tender. Smash a few lentils with your finger to test. Cook a bit longer if any are firm in the middle.

3. Remove the bay leaf. Process in a food processor until smooth. Thin with water as needed. Season with salt and lemon juice.

4. Spread into a shallow bowl and top with the diced onions. Serve with sliced vegetables or pita chips.

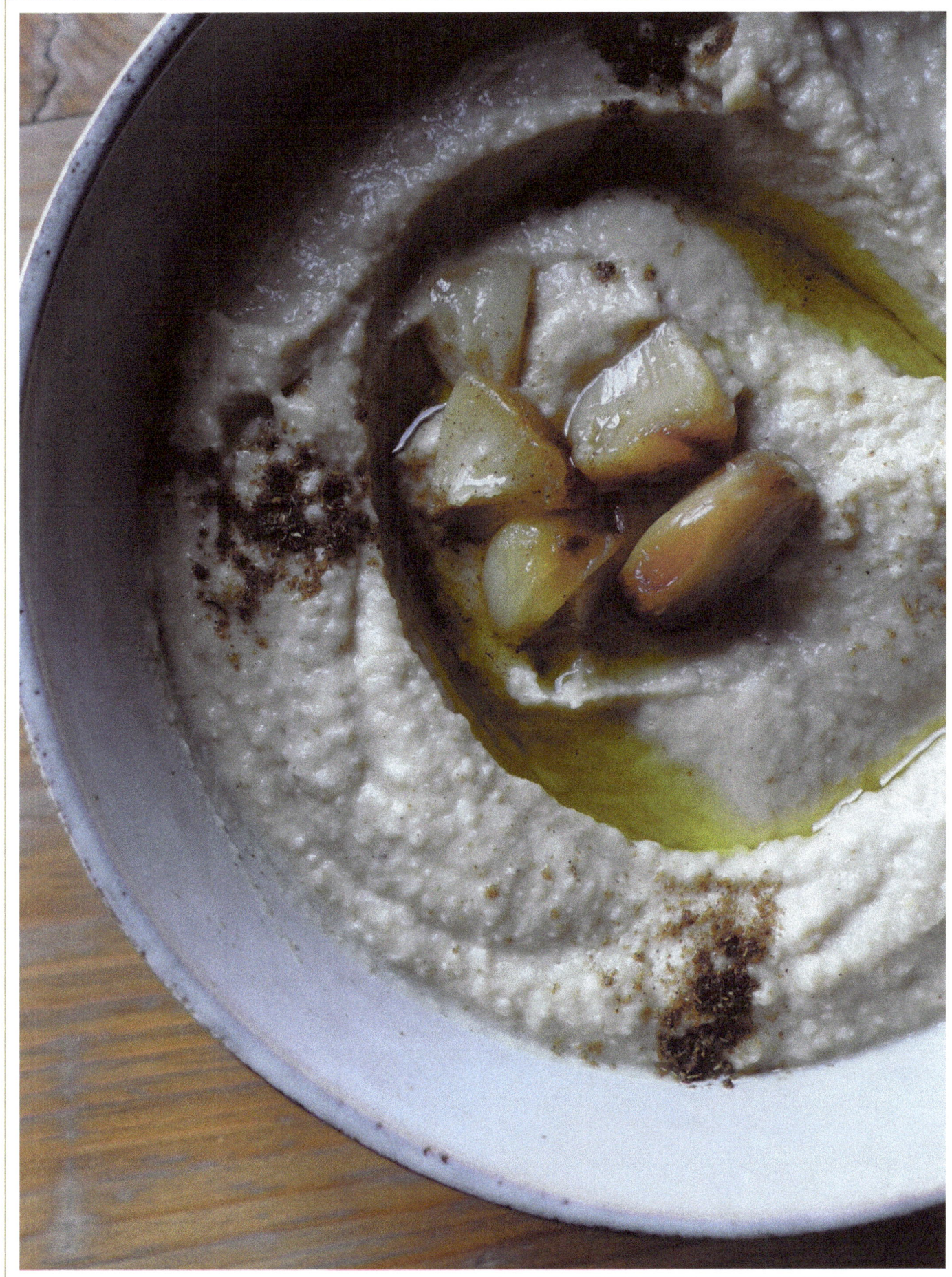

HUMMUS

Ancient people loved hummus as much as we do today! The earliest recipe was discovered in a 13th century cookbook from Cairo, Egypt. This simple formula yields silky smooth results every time.

Prepare the Chickpeas

1 lb. (16-oz.) dried chickpeas, rinsed
2 tsp. baking soda (to soak)
water

If making a half batch of hummus, freeze half of the cooked chickpeas for next time. Or just cook half of the bag (8-oz.) instead of the full pound.

1. Soak dried chickpeas overnight with baking soda and enough water to cover by a few inches.

2. Drain and rinse the chickpeas the next day. Boil in fresh water for an hour or until the chickpeas are super soft. *To test carefully remove a few chickpeas with a slotted spoon and smash on a plate. Are all of your test chickpeas velvety smooth? If not, keep boiling to avoid gritty hummus.

3. Drain the chickpeas. (Freeze half if making a half batch. Or make soup with the rest!)

Make Hummus!

Choose a recipe from the next page. Process the ingredients in a food processor until ultra smooth. Thin with water as needed. Season to taste with lemon juice and sea salt. Cover and refrigerate for an hour before serving. Serve with a splash of good extra-virgin olive oil.

CLASSIC HUMMUS

Full Batch

6 cups cooked chickpeas
(total yield from 1 lb. bag)
½ cup fresh lemon juice
½ cup tahini sesame paste
2 garlic cloves, peeled
1 tsp. ground cumin
sea salt, to taste

Half Batch

3 cups cooked chickpeas or 2 (15-oz.) cans cooked chickpeas, drained and rinsed
¼ cup fresh lemon juice
¼ cup tahini sesame paste
1 garlic clove, peeled
½ tsp. ground cumin
sea salt, to taste

Red Pepper Hummus (Small Batch)

1½ cups cooked chickpeas or 1 (15-oz.) can cooked chickpeas, drained and rinsed
½ cup roasted red peppers (from the jar or home-roasted and peeled)
2 Tbsp. tahini sesame paste
1 garlic clove, peeled
1 tsp. paprika (or try smoked paprika)
½ tsp. cayenne pepper, or more to taste
lemon juice, to taste
sea salt, to taste
water (to thin)

Black Olive Hummus (Small Batch)

1½ cups cooked chickpeas or 1 (15-oz.) can cooked chickpeas, drained and rinsed
½ cup pitted black olives
¼ cup pitted Kalamata olives
2 Tbsp. tahini sesame paste
1 garlic clove, peeled
lemon juice, to taste
sea salt, to taste
water (to thin)

Pickled Beet Hummus (Small Batch)

1½ cups cooked chickpeas or 1 (15-oz.) can cooked chickpeas, drained and rinsed
¾ cup chopped pickled beets (or peeled boiled or roasted beets)
2 Tbsp. tahini sesame paste
1 garlic clove, peeled
lemon juice, to taste
½ tsp. lemon zest
sea salt, to taste
water (to thin)

Jalapeno Hummus (Small Batch)

2 jalapenos
extra-virgin olive oil
1½ cups cooked chickpeas or 1 (15-oz.) can cooked chickpeas, drained and rinsed
¼ cup cilantro leaves, lightly packed
2 Tbsp. tahini sesame paste
1 garlic clove, peeled
½ tsp. ground cumin
lemon juice, to taste
sea salt, to taste
water (to thin)

1. Preheat your oven to 425°F. Rub the peppers with olive oil. Roast for 30 minutes on a parchment-lined sheet pan. Flip once halfway through cooking.
2. Transfer the peppers to an airtight container or resealable plastic bag. Let the peppers steam for 15 minutes. Then peel off as much skin as you can. Remove the stems and scrape out the seeds.
3. Place the jalapenos into a food processor with the rest of the ingredients. Process until very smooth. Thin with water as needed.

Roasted Garlic Hummus (Small Batch)

1 entire head of garlic (use two if they're small)
extra-virgin olive oil
1½ cups cooked chickpeas or 1 (15-oz.) can cooked chickpeas, drained and rinsed
¼ cup tahini sesame paste
½ tsp. ground cumin
lemon juice, to taste
sea salt, to taste
water (to thin)

1. Roast the garlic: Preheat your oven to 400°F. Slice off the top of the garlic to expose as many cloves as possible. Coat the garlic with olive oil and wrap it in foil. Roast for 45 minutes.
2. Set the garlic aside to cool. Unwrap it and squeeze the tender cloves into a food processor with its root-end in your palm. The cloves should pop out easily.
3. Add the rest of the ingredients and process until very smooth. Thin with water if needed.

APPETIZERS

Marinated Mushrooms

Marinated Feta & Olives

Feta & Watermelon

Grilled Prosciutto & Cantaloupe Skewers

Garden Kebabs

Lemon & Spice Pork Pinchitos

Lamb Arrosticini with Mint Gremolata

Honey Dill Salmon Brochettes

Roasted Cauliflower Bites
with Jalapeno Tahini Dip

Turkish Hot Wings

Greek Meatballs with Feta Mousse

Marinated Mushrooms

Graze on these with other antipasti, charcuterie, or straight from the fridge when on the go.

8 oz. small white or cremini mushrooms, cleaned
water (to boil)
¼ cup extra-virgin olive oil
3 Tbsp. red wine vinegar
2 Tbsp. chopped flat-leaf parsley
3 garlic cloves, minced
½ tsp. dried oregano
¼ tsp. red pepper flakes
freshly ground black pepper, to taste
sea salt, to taste

    1. Leave small mushrooms whole. Cut large ones in half or quarters. Boil in salted water for 5 minutes. Drain and rinse with cold water. Pat dry.
    2. Combine remaining ingredients in a non-reactive container with a lid. Add mushrooms and mix well. (Also add some artichokes, olives, or peppers if you'd like.)
    3. Cover and marinate four hours or overnight, stirring occasionally. Serve at room temperature.

Marinated Feta & Olives

¼ cup extra-virgin olive oil
1 lemon, juice and zest
1 garlic clove, minced
2 tsp. fresh thyme leaves, chopped (or ½ tsp. dried thyme)
½ tsp. dried oregano
½ tsp. freshly ground black pepper
½ tsp. red pepper flakes
8 oz.. brined feta cheese block
¼ cup pitted green olives
¼ cup pitted Kalamata olives
accompaniment: crackers or toasted bread (e.g., crostini)

1. Mix the oil, lemon, garlic, and seasonings in a resealable container.
2. Cut feta into small cubes. Add feta and olives to the marinade. Lightly toss. Refrigerate four hours or overnight, stirring occasionally.

Feta & Watermelon

Ancient Egyptians prized the watermelon for its high water content. Pair the sweet fruit with salty feta for a hydrating beach snack or summer party appetizer.

1 ripe seedless watermelon
  (Look for a golden creamy spot.
   It's had time to ripen in the field.)
6-8 oz. block feta
fresh mint leaves (optional)

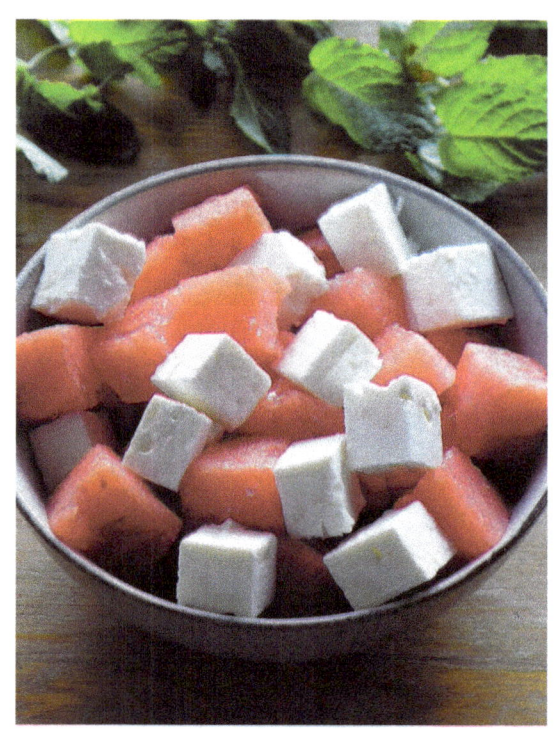

Serving Ideas

- Graze on a platter of sliced melon and feta that are side-by-side.
- Place diced melon into a serving dish and crumble with feta like a salad.
- Layer onto small bamboo picks; diced feta, mint leaf, then diced melon.

Grilled Prosciutto & Cantaloupe Skewers

8 bamboo skewers
1 cantaloupe, balled or cubed
4 oz. (about 8 slices) prosciutto, torn into pieces
sea salt
freshly ground black pepper, to taste
balsamic glaze (optional)

Variation

Skip the grill and serve chilled. Add a few spearmint or basil leaves to each skewer.

1. First soak your skewers in water for at least 30 minutes to avoid burnt skewers.
2. String melon balls onto each skewer. Fold a few ribbons of prosciutto onto each skewer here and there. Lightly dust with sea salt and black pepper
3. Grill for about 2 minutes on each side until charred. Drizzle with balsamic just before serving.

Garden Kebabs

8 bamboo skewers (soaked in water for 30 minutes)
1 lb. (16-oz.) medium white or cremini button mushrooms
1 pint cherry tomatoes
1 zucchini, cut into ½-inch-thick rounds
¼ cup extra-virgin olive oil
1 Tbsp. minced fresh parsley
1 Tbsp. chopped fresh thyme leaves
3 garlic cloves, crushed into a paste
sea salt and freshly ground black pepper, to taste

1. Trim ends and wipe mushrooms clean with a paper towel. Don't rinse – mushrooms absorb liquid like a sponge. String a pattern of mushrooms, tomatoes, and zucchini onto each skewer. Place onto a baking sheet in a single layer.
2. Combine the oil, parsley, thyme, and garlic. Generously brush onto each skewer. Season well with salt and pepper.
3. Grill over medium-high heat 8-10 minutes, turning occasionally. Alternatively, roast for 15-20 minutes on a parchment-lined baking sheet in an oven preheated to 425F. Transfer to a serving platter and serve immediately.

Lemon & Spice Pork Pinchitos

Marinade
¼ cup extra-virgin olive oil
1 lemon, juice and zest
2 garlic cloves, crushed into a paste
1 tsp. paprika
1 tsp. ground cumin
1 tsp. ground coriander
1 tsp. dried thyme
1 tsp. fine sea salt
½ tsp smoked paprika
¼ tsp. black pepper
¼ tsp. cinnamon
¼ tsp. turmeric

8 bamboo or metal skewers
1 lb. boneless pork tenderloin, cut into ¾-inch cubes
(substitute: chicken or lamb)
bread loaf, such as Italian bread, diagonally sliced 1-inch

Accompaniments
lemon wedges (to finish)
handful chopped cilantro (to garnish)
glass of wine (optional)

1. Combine marinade ingredients in a resealable plastic bag or container. Pat the meat dry and add to the bag. Coat with the marinade. Refrigerate two hours or overnight for the best flavor.

2. Soak wooden skewers for 30 minutes in water. Let the meat come to room temperature on the counter too.

3. Thread meat onto skewers slightly spaced apart. Then thickly slice the bread and wrap the entire loaf in foil.

4. To Grill: Place the bread loaf onto the coolest part of your grill to warm. Grill pinchitos over medium-high heat until cooked thoroughly, turning a few times (6-10 minutes). Let the pork rest for five minutes.

5. Squeeze lemon over your pinchitos and sprinkle with cilantro. Slide meat off skewers with warm bread. Serve with wine and lemon wedges.

Lamb Arrosticini with Mint Gremolata

¼ cup fresh mint leaves
¼ cup flat-leaf parsley leaves
¼ cup extra-virgin olive oil
1 tsp. lemon zest
1 garlic clove, peeled
Pinch of sea salt

8 bamboo skewers (soak in water for at least 30 minutes)
1 lb. boneless lamb, cut into ¾ x ½-inch cubes
¼ cup extra-virgin olive oil
1 long rosemary sprig (to brush)
Sea salt and black pepper
Sliced bread

1. <u>For the Gremolata</u>: Blend mint, parsley, oil, zest, garlic, and salt in a small food processor. Set aside.
2. Thread the lamb onto the skewers tightly. Grill over medium-high heat for about 5 minutes, turning occasionally. Grill the bread if desired.
3. Transfer to a clean plate. Use the rosemary sprig to brush extra-virgin olive oil all over the hot arrosticini. Season with salt and pepper. Enjoy arrosticini on bread with a dollop of gremolata.

Honey Dill Salmon Brochettes

Honey Dill Marinade

¼ cup extra-virgin olive oil

2 Tbsp. honey

2 Tbsp. chopped fresh dill (plus more to garnish)

1 Tbsp. fresh lemon juice

½ tsp. minced garlic

½ tsp. Dijon mustard

½ tsp. fine sea salt

1 lb. skinless salmon, cut into 1-inch cubes

8 bamboo skewers (soaked in water for at least 30 minutes)

1 lemon, sliced thin (optional)

1. Whisk together the marinade ingredients in a large bowl. Add the salmon and mix well to coat. Let sit for 20 minutes. Thread the salmon and lemon onto skewers in a pattern.

2. Grill over medium heat for 6-8 minutes with the lid closed, flipping once. Garnish with fresh dill.

Roasted Cauliflower Bites with Jalapeno Tahini Dip

Jalapeno Tahini Dip

½ cup tahini sesame paste
¼ cup water
¼ cup fresh lemon juice
¼ cup (packed) chopped cilantro (plus more to garnish)
1 jalapeno, cored
2 garlic cloves, peeled
½ tsp. fine sea salt, or more to taste

2 Tbsp. extra-virgin olive oil
½ tsp. ground cumin
sea salt and freshly ground black pepper, to taste
1 large head cauliflower

1. Blend dip ingredients in a small food processor until smooth. Thin with water as needed. Reserve.
2. Preheat oven to 400°F. Cut cauliflower into florets. Toss with oil, cumin, salt, and pepper. Space apart on a baking sheet. Roast 15-25 minutes or until fork tender.
3. Pour dip into a small bowl for dipping or drizzle it onto the cauliflower instead. Garnish with additional cilantro.

Turkish Hot Wings

¼ cup extra-virgin olive oil
¼ cup plain whole milk yogurt
2 Tbsp. tomato paste
1 Tbsp. fresh lemon juice
3 garlic cloves, minced
2 tsp. paprika
1 tsp. cayenne pepper
1 tsp. dried oregano
1 tsp. fine sea salt
½ tsp. smoked paprika
½ tsp. black pepper
2 lb. chicken wings (or drumsticks)

1. Whisk together the marinade ingredients in a large bowl. Pat the wings or drumsticks dry and coat with the marinade. Cover and refrigerate 4 hours or overnight.
2. 30 minutes prior to cooking, line a pan with parchment or an oiled oven-safe rack. Arrange a layer of chicken and bring to room temperature on the counter.
3. Preheat your oven to 400°F. Bake for 25-35 minutes (35-40 minutes for drumsticks) or until juices run clear and the minimum internal temperature is 180°F.

Greek Meatballs with Feta Mousse

This lifestyle isn't about strict rules. So if you consume lean red meat on occasion—enjoy every guilt-free bite. These meatballs are traditional Greek mezze. So savor a few with feta mousse or tzatziki.

Feta Mousse
½ cup Greek yogurt (or freshly home-strained)
½ cup (4-oz.) brined feta cheese, roughly chopped

Meatballs
1 Tbsp. extra-virgin olive oil
½ cup diced onion
sea salt
1 garlic clove, minced
¼ tsp. red pepper flakes
1 egg
½ cup milk
2 Tbsp. minced parsley
1 Tbsp. fresh spearmint leaves, chopped (or 1 tsp. dried spearmint)
1 tsp. dried oregano
1 tsp. sea salt

½ tsp. black pepper

⅛ tsp. baking soda

½ cup quick-cooking oats (or breadcrumbs)

1 lb. lean ground beef
  (or use a combination of lean beef, pork, and/or lamb)

lemon wedges (to serve)

Variation

Dice a block of brined feta cheese into small cubes. Push a cube of feta into each meatball when forming. Reseal the opening. Bake as directed.

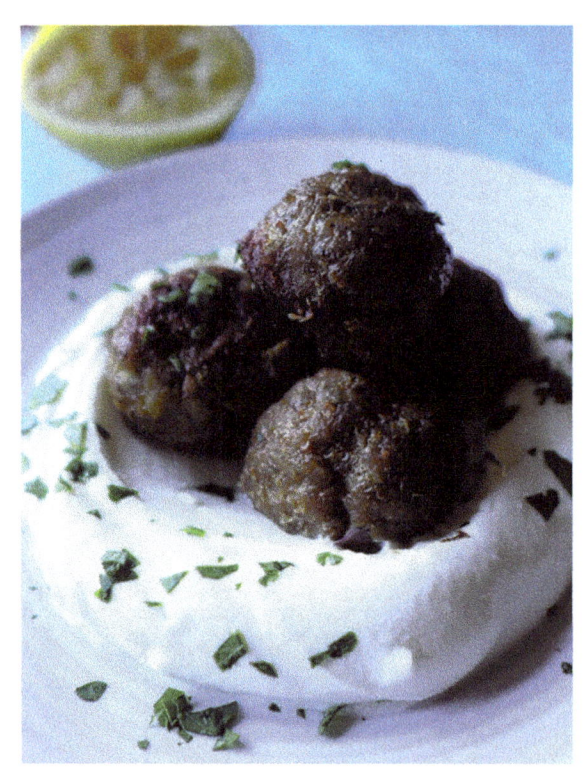

1. <u>Feta Mousse</u>: Blend ingredients in a small food processor until smooth and whipped, scraping down the sides.

2. <u>Meatballs</u>: Heat the olive oil in a pan. Cook the onions until soft with a good pinch of salt. Add the garlic and red pepper flakes. Cook for two more minutes. Turn off the heat and set aside to cool.

3. Combine the egg, milk, herbs, seasonings, and baking soda in a large bowl. Add the oats, meat, and onion mixture. Mix thoroughly, but don't overmix.

4. Preheat the oven to 400°F. Line a sheet pan with parchment. Form 1½-inch meatballs and space apart on the pan. Bake on the center rack for 20 minutes, or until cooked throughout.

5. Squeeze lemon over the meatballs. Serve with lemon wedges and feta mousse.

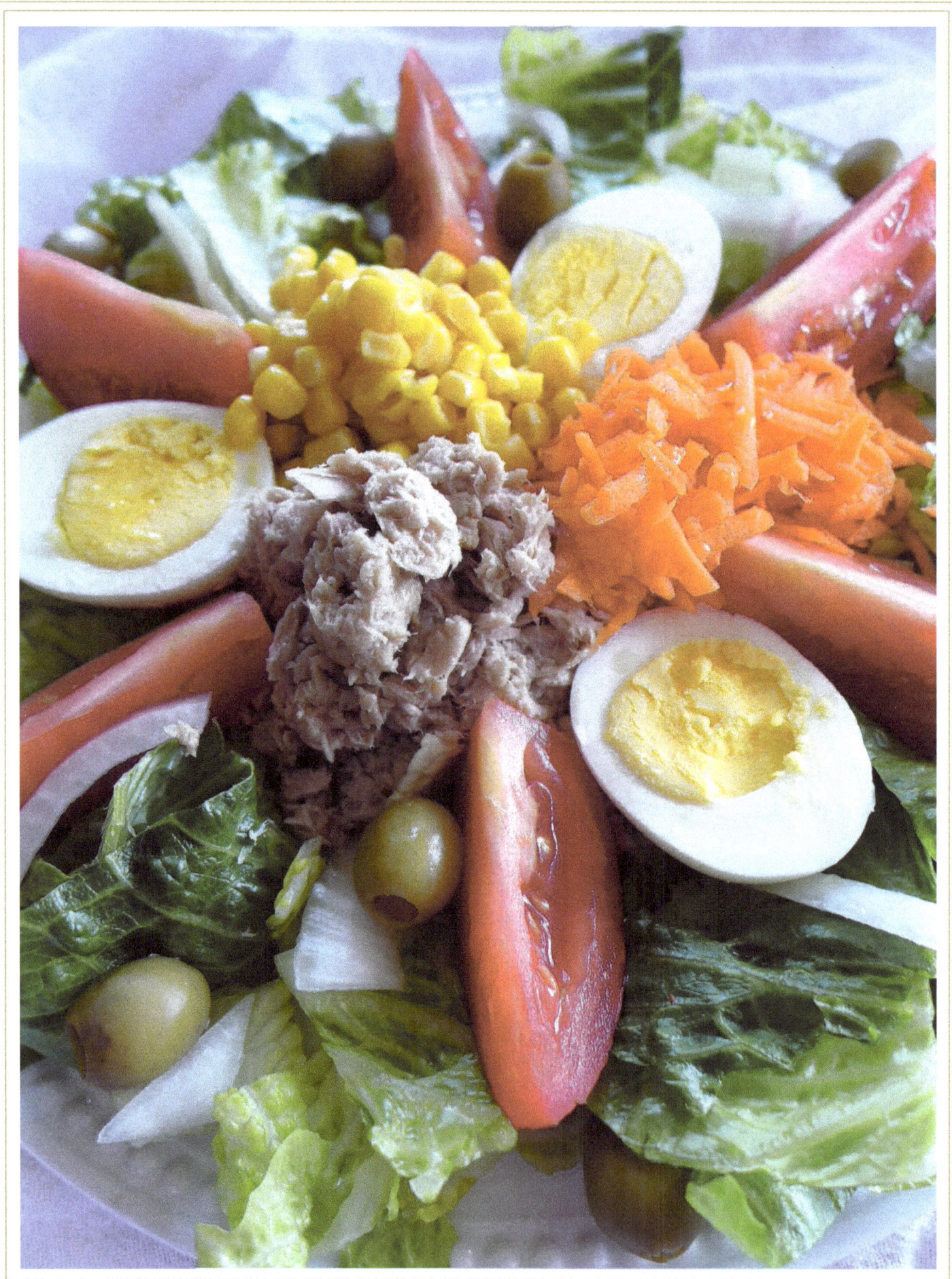

SALADS

Baked Croutons

Honey Roasted Nuts

Sea Salt Roasted Chickpeas

Roasted Eggplant Cubes

Salad Bar Chicken

Simple Flaked Salmon

Egyptian Smashed Feta & Cucumber Salad

Moroccan Tomato & Cucumber Salad

Whole Grain Tabouli

Balela Bean Salad

Cannellini Tuna Salad with Fried Capers

Black-Eyed Pea Tuna Salad

Summer Berry Salad with Balsamic Vinaigrette

Italian Chicken Sub Salad

Arugula & Parmesan Salad

Aegean Herb Salad with Greek Feta Dressing

Valencian Salad

Poached Salmon Niçoise

with Old Style Mustard Vinaigrette

Baked Croutons

5 cups diced bread
 (Stale is fine.)
3 Tbsp. extra-virgin olive oil
½ tsp. black pepper
½ tsp. garlic powder
¼ tsp. fine sea salt

1. Preheat your oven to 325°F. Whisk together the olive oil and seasonings in a large bowl. Add the bread and toss well to coat. Space apart on a sheet pan.

2. Bake for 15 minutes. Rotate the pan and bake another 15 minutes. Set aside to cool completely. Store at room temperature in an air-tight container.

Honey Roasted Nuts

3 Tbsp. honey (or pure maple syrup)
2 tsp. extra-virgin olive oil
¼ tsp. cinnamon (or use cayenne instead for spicy hot honey nuts)
¼ tsp. sea salt
1 cup nuts (whole or halved; walnuts, pecans, or almonds)

1. Preheat your oven to 325°F. Line a rimmed sheet pan with parchment. Lightly oil the parchment. Whisk the honey, oil, cinnamon and/or cayenne, and salt in a large bowl. Add nuts and mix well.
2. Spread nuts onto the pan in a single layer. Bake 10-20 minutes or until toasted, stirring occasionally.
3. Set aside to cool completely before handling. Hot sugar is super dangerous. Store at room temperature in an airtight container.

Sea Salt Roasted Chickpeas

1 (15-oz.) can chickpeas, drained and rinsed
1 tsp. extra-virgin olive oil
¼ tsp. fine sea salt

1. Preheat your oven to 350°F. Rub chickpeas completely dry with paper towel. Discard loosened skins.
2. Mix the chickpeas, oil, and salt in a bowl. Bake for 30 minutes on a sheet pan. Turn off the oven, but leave the chickpeas in for another 30 minutes to crisp.
3. Remove from the oven and set aside to cool completely. Store in an airtight container at room temperature.

Roasted Eggplant Cubes

1 medium eggplant, diced 1-inch
2 Tbsp. extra-virgin olive oil
sea salt and black pepper, to taste

1. Preheat your oven to 425°F. Line a sheet pan with parchment otherwise the eggplant will stick to the pan.
2. Pile the cubes onto the pan and drizzle with olive oil. Season with salt and pepper. Toss well. Space cubes apart.
3. Bake for 30 minutes. Rotate the pan after 15 minutes. Remove and set aside to cool. Snack on these anytime, or toss into salads, sandwiches, pasta, or omelets.

Salad Bar Chicken

Roast a few boneless chicken breasts in advance for easy, healthy meals later. Toss into leafy green salads, pasta, vegetable skillets, and more.

1 lb. (2 to 3) boneless, skinless chicken breasts
2 Tbsp. extra-virgin olive oil
1 lemon, juiced
2 tsp. dried oregano, thyme, or parsley (optional)
¾ tsp. sea salt
½ tsp. freshly ground black pepper
1 garlic clove, crushed into a paste (or ½ tsp. granulated garlic)

1. Preheat the oven to 425°F. Line a sheet pan with parchment for easy clean-up.
2. Pound chicken to an even thickness between two sheets of plastic wrap or in a large resealable plastic bag. Larger breasts can be cut horizontally to make two cutlets before pounding to an even thickness.
3. Whisk the rest of the ingredients in a large bowl (or resealable plastic bag). Add chicken and coat with the mixture. Marinate 30 minutes on the counter.

4. Arrange the chicken on the pan. Bake 15-25 minutes or until it reaches a safe internal temperature of 165°F at its thickest part.

5. Rest 5-10 minutes before cutting. Slice against the grain, dice, or shred the chicken. Refrigerate or freeze until ready to use.

Simple Flaked Salmon

Prepare salmon in advance for a quick boost of omega-3 fatty acids. Scatter flakes over green salads and bean salads, toss with rice and vegetables, or whip up a decadent seafood pasta.

2 to 4 (6-oz.) salmon fillets, skin-on
extra-virgin olive oil
sea salt, to taste
freshly ground black pepper, to taste

1. Preheat your oven to 400°F. Line a sheet pan with parchment. Pat salmon dry. Lightly coat with oil and season with salt and pepper. Arrange skin-side down on the pan. Let the salmon come to room temperature for 30 minutes on the counter.

2. Bake 12-15 minutes or until salmon flakes easily with a fork. Let rest for 10 minutes. Refrigerate until ready to use. Beware of small bones. Flake chunks of salmon with a fork and use as desired.

Egyptian Smashed Feta & Cucumber Salad

½ cup (4-oz.) brined feta cheese, crumbled
2 Tbsp. extra-virgin olive oil
2 Tbsp. fresh lemon juice
1 English seedless cucumber, diced
½ cup finely diced red onion (substitute: scallions)
1 Tbsp. minced fresh mint leaves (substitute: parsley or dill)
sea salt and freshly ground black pepper

1. Place feta, oil, and lemon into a large bowl. Smash together with a fork.
2. Add the cucumbers, onions, and herbs. Season to taste with salt and pepper.

Moroccan Tomato & Cucumber Salad

½ cucumber, peeled and diced
2 Roma tomatoes, cored and diced   (optionally peeled)
¼ cup finely diced red onion
2 Tbsp. minced flat-leaf parsley
splash extra-virgin olive oil
splash red wine vinegar (or lemon)
freshly ground black pepper
sea salt

1. Combine ingredients. Season to taste with vinegar, pepper, and salt. Marinate for at least 30 minutes before serving.

Whole Grain Tabouli

½ cup fine bulgur wheat (#1) (or 1 cup prepared quinoa)
pinch sea salt (plus more for the salad)
1 cup boiling water

¼ cup extra-virgin olive oil
1 lemon, juiced
1 garlic clove, minced
1 bunch curly parsley, finely chopped
2 Roma tomatoes, finely diced
½ cup diced cucumber (optional)
½ cup sliced scallions
2 Tbsp. chopped fresh mint
freshly ground black pepper

1. Place bulgur and salt into a bowl. Pour in the boiling water and stir. Cover and set aside for 12 minutes. The bulgur will absorb most of the water. Pour into a fine mesh strainer to remove excess moisture. Set aside.
2. Mix the olive oil, lemon, garlic, parsley, tomatoes, cucumber, scallions, and mint in a large bowl. Toss in; the bulgur and season to taste with salt and pepper. Mix well. Refrigerate for one hour before serving.

Balela Bean Salad

¼ cup extra-virgin olive oil
1 lemon, juiced (plus ½ tsp. lemon zest)
1 garlic clove, minced
½ tsp. sea salt, or to taste
freshly ground black pepper, to taste
pinch red pepper flakes

1 (15-oz.) can chickpeas, drained and rinsed
1 (15-oz.) can black beans, drained and rinsed
2 Roma tomatoes, cored and diced small (or 1 cup halved cherry tomatoes)
¼ cup sliced Kalamata or green olives (or a mixture)
¼ cup finely diced red onion
¼ cup chopped parsley leaves
2 Tbsp. chopped fresh mint

    1. Combine olive oil, lemon, garlic, salt, pepper, and red pepper flakes in a large bowl.
    2. Add the beans, tomatoes, olives, onions, and herbs. Mix well. Add more salt, pepper, or lemon juice if needed. Refrigerate for one hour before serving.

Cannellini Tuna Salad with Fried Capers

Crispy fried capers elevate this traditional Tuscan salad.

Fried Capers
¼ cup capers
¼ cup extra-virgin olive oil

1 (15-oz.) can cannellini beans, drained and rinsed
1 small red onion, thinly sliced
2 Tbsp. chopped Italian flat-leaf parsleyN
3 Tbsp. extra-virgin olive oil (plus more to drizzle)
1 Tbsp. red wine vinegar
sea salt and black pepper, to taste
1 (5-oz.) can albacore or chunk light tuna, drained

*Optionally toss with some artichoke hearts, black olives, or a cup of cooked pasta.

1. <u>Fry the capers</u>: Pat the capers completely dry with a paper towel. Heat the oil in a small pot until it shimmers. Test one caper. If it sizzles the oil is ready. Pour in the rest of the capers and fry until lightly browned and puffed open (this can take seconds or up to three minutes). Remove with a slotted spoon and drain on paper towel. Reserve.

2. <u>For the salad</u>: Combine the beans, onions, parsley, olive oil, and vinegar in a large bowl. Season with salt and pepper. Mix well. Add the tuna and gently toss, leaving larger chunks intact. Drizzle with extra-virgin olive oil when serving and scatter with fried capers.

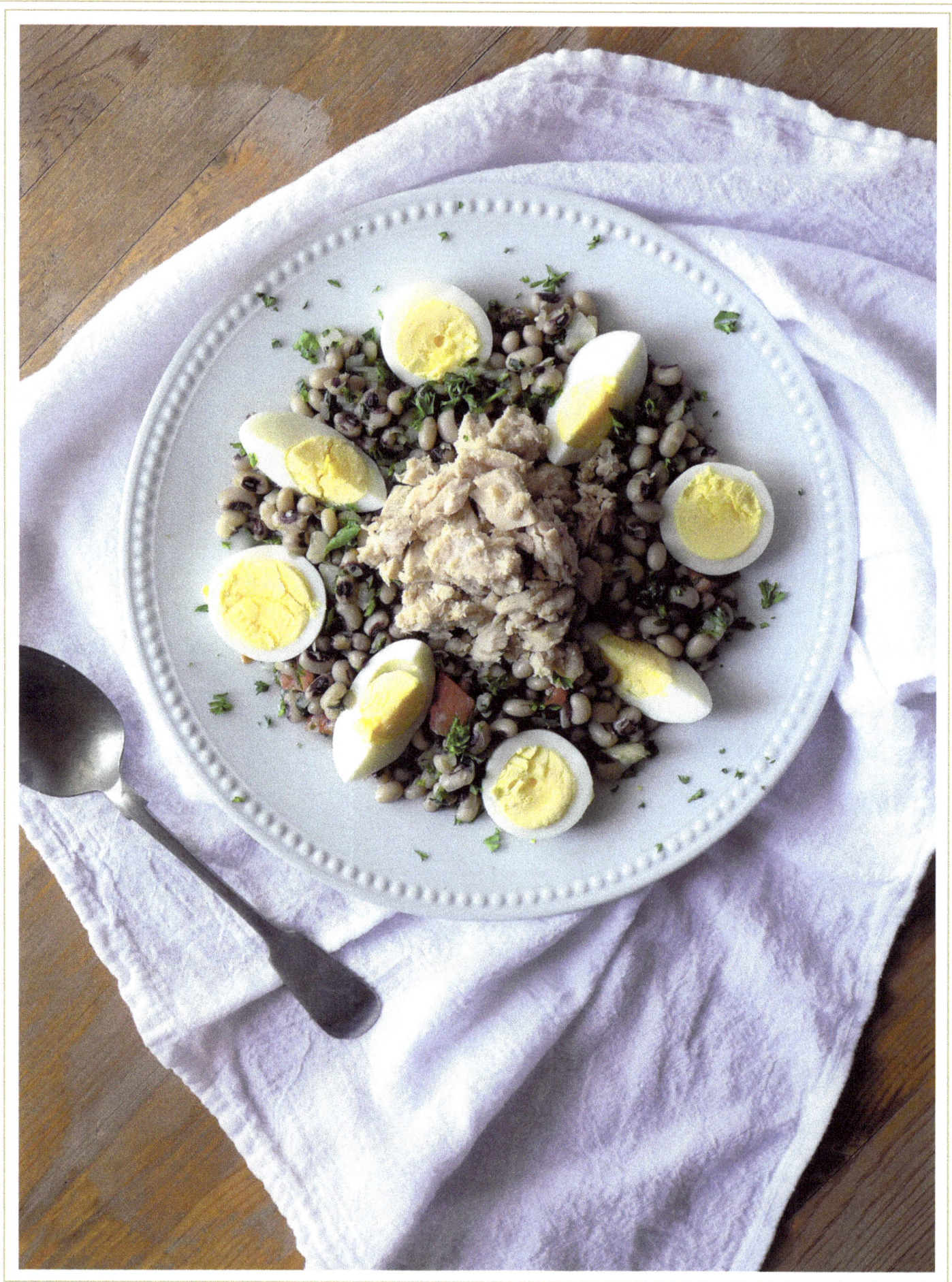

Black-Eyed Pea Tuna Salad

1 (15-oz.) can black-eyed peas, drained and rinsed
½ cup diced white onion
¼ cup chopped cilantro
3 Tbsp. extra-virgin olive oil
2 Tbsp. white wine vinegar
1 garlic clove, minced
sea salt and black pepper, to taste
1 (5-oz.) can albacore or chunk light tuna, drained
handful of black or green olives
2 hard-boiled eggs, halved, quartered, or chopped

1. Toss together the black-eyed peas, onions, cilantro, olive oil, vinegar, and garlic in a large bowl. Season with salt and pepper.
2. Before serving add the tuna and lightly toss – or top with a scoop instead. Garnish with olives and eggs.

Summer Berry Salad with Balsamic Vinaigrette

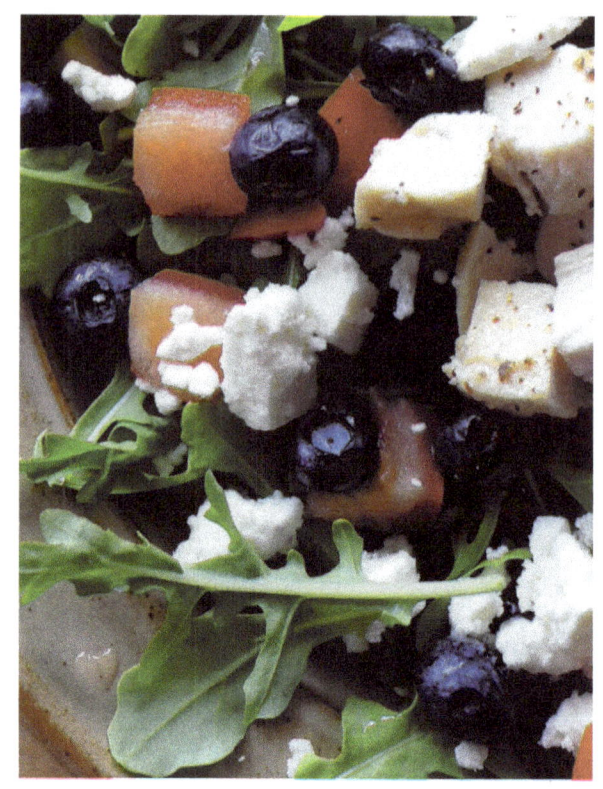

Balsamic Vinaigrette
3 Tbsp. extra-virgin olive oil
1 Tbsp. balsamic vinegar
1 Tbsp. lemon juice
1 tsp. honey
sea salt, to taste
black pepper, to taste

1 cup fresh mixed berries
4 cups mixed baby greens, baby spinach, or baby arugula
1 cup diced cooked chicken (optional)
¼ cup (2-oz.) crumbled feta or goat cheese
¼ cup chopped almonds, walnuts, pepitas, or sunflower seeds

1. For the dressing: Combine ingredients in a jar. Cover and shake well. Feel free to use balsamic glaze instead or just splash some balsamic and extra-virgin olive oil.
2. Just before serving toss the berries, greens, and chicken with just enough dressing to coat. Sprinkle the cheese and nuts/seeds on top.

Italian Chicken Sub Salad

This salad is doused with herby Sub Sauce for maximum Italian Sub flavor. We replace the usual cold-cuts with lean chicken or plant-based chickpeas.

Sub Sauce

6 Tbsp. extra-virgin olive oil
¼ cup red wine vinegar
1½ tsp. dried oregano
½ tsp. dried basil
¼ tsp. freshly ground black pepper
¼ tsp. garlic powder
¼ tsp. sea salt, or to taste

1 small head iceberg lettuce, shredded
1 cup diced cooked chicken (or chickpeas)
1 cup cherry tomatoes, halved
½ medium red onion, thinly sliced
½ cup diced or sliced provolone
½ cup black olives
⅓ cup sliced peperoncini
1 cup croutons (optional)

1. <u>Sub Sauce</u>: Combine ingredients in jar. Cover and shake well.

2. <u>Salad</u>: Layer the ingredients in a large serving bowl. Toss with just enough Sub Sauce to coat the salad just before serving.

Cheat-Day Variation
Add ½ cup chopped ham and ½ cup chopped salami.

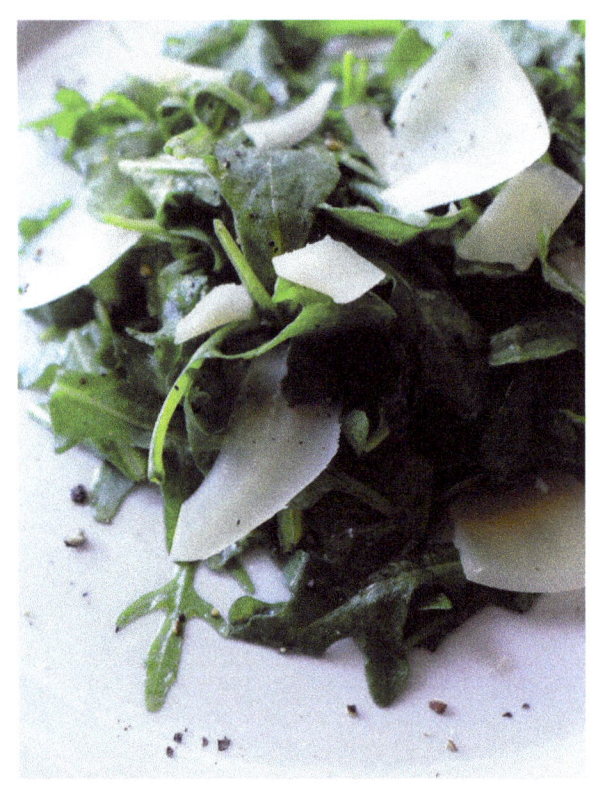

Arugula & Parmesan Salad

Arugula has been considered a potent aphrodesiac since ancient times and was once forbidden from monastic gardens. Keep some in stock to whip up this beautifully simple snack or starter.

a handful of arugula
fresh lemon juice, to taste (alternatively: balsamic vinegar)
splash extra-virgin olive oil
sea salt, to taste
freshly ground black pepper, to taste
wedge Parmigiano-Reggiano

1. Place a handful of arugula onto a plate. Squeeze with lemon and splash with olive oil.
2. Season with salt and pepper. Shave petals of Parmigiano-Reggiano over the salad.

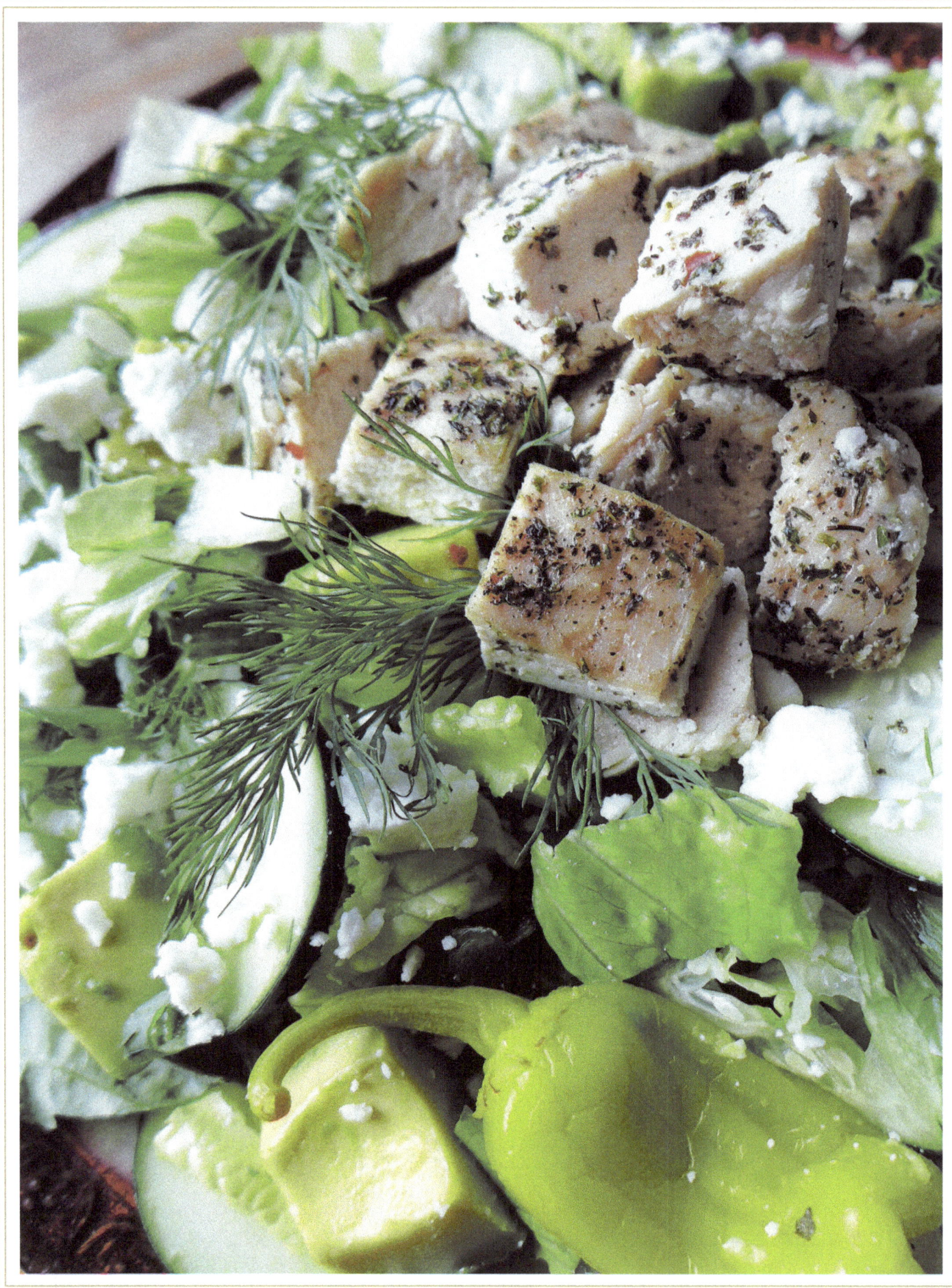

Aegean Herb Salad with Greek Feta Dressing

Greek Feta Dressing
6 Tbsp. extra-virgin olive oil
2 Tbsp. red wine vinegar
2 Tbsp. brined feta cheese, smashed
1 Tbsp. fresh lemon juice
1 tsp. dried oregano
½ tsp. minced garlic
½ tsp. fine sea salt
freshly ground black pepper, to taste

1 large head romaine lettuce, chopped
½ cucumber, cut lengthwise and sliced
½ cup sliced scallions
¼ cup fresh dill, chopped
1 cup cooked chickpeas or diced chicken (optional)
½ cup (4-oz.) brined feta cheese
¼ cup sliced peperoncini peppers
¼ cup Kalamata olives

1. For the dressing: Combine ingredients in a jar. Cover and shake well. Reserve.
2. Place the romaine, cucumbers, scallions, and dill into a large bowl. Toss with just enough dressing to coat.

3. Optionally add chickpeas or chicken. Top with crumbled feta cheese, peperoncini, and olives. Serve immediately.

Valencian Salad

Dressed simply with sea salt and olive oil, this Spanish salad is served family-style.

½ head iceberg lettuce, chopped (or a head of romaine)
2 Roma tomatoes, sliced
1 small white onion, sliced
½ cup shredded carrots (optional)
½ cup corn kernels
sea salt, to taste
1 (5-oz.) can tuna (preferably packed in oil), drained
½ cup pitted green olives
2 hard-boiled eggs, halved
1 avocado, pitted and quartered
extra-virgin olive oil

*A few spears of white asparagus are sometimes added in Spain, where it's a delicacy.

1. Place a bed of lettuce onto a serving platter. Arrange a layer of tomatoes. Sprinkle a layer of onions, then carrots, and finally corn.

2. Season with pinches of sea salt.

3. Place a few chunks of tuna onto the salad. Scatter the green olives. Then garnish with the eggs and avocado, if using.

4. Generously drizzle some good extra-virgin olive oil all over the salad. Enjoy!

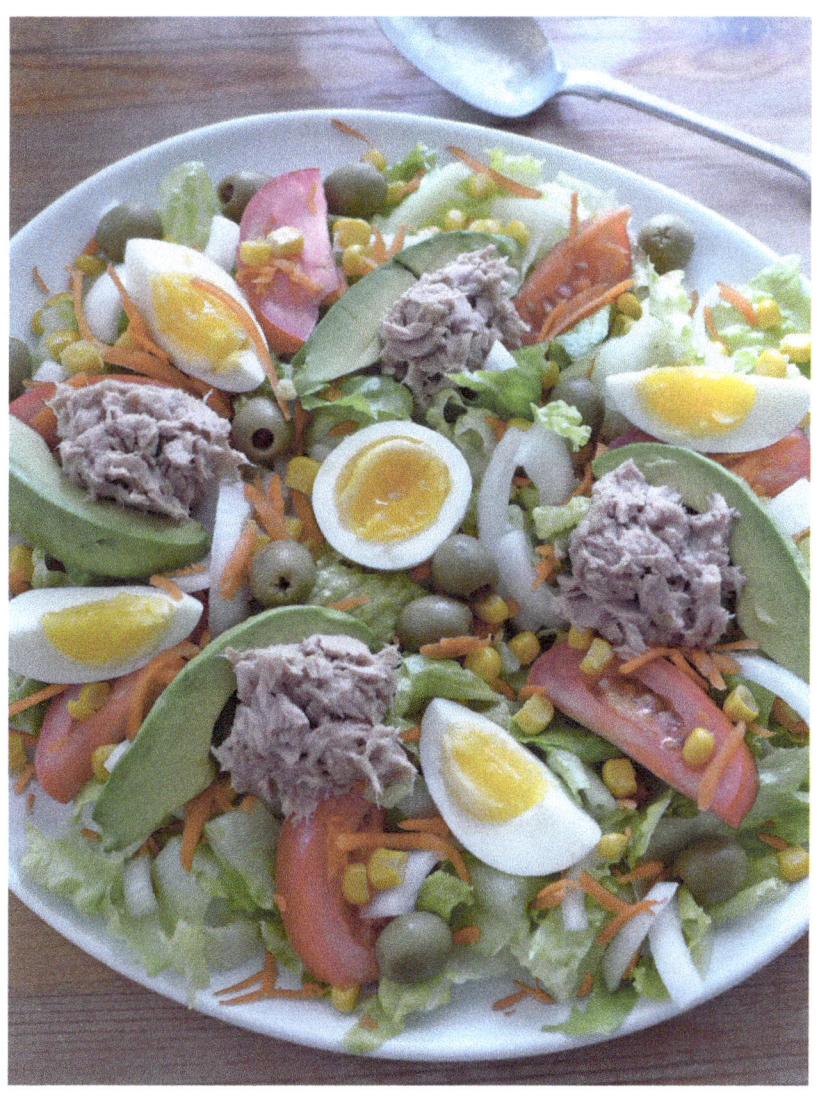

Poached Salmon Niçoise with Old Style Mustard Vinaigrette

Old Style Mustard Vinaigrette

¼ cup extra-virgin olive oil

1½ Tbsp. apple cider vinegar

1 Tbsp. whole grain mustard

1 tsp. honey

sea salt and freshly ground black pepper, to taste

Poached Salmon

(substitute: 1 (5-oz.) can tuna in oil, a few anchovies, or leftover baked salmon)

1 lemon, sliced

1½ tsp. sea salt

½ tsp. peppercorns (or coarsely ground pepper)

2 skinless salmon fillets

water (enough to cover the salmon)

4-8 oz. thin green beans or haricot verts, trimmed (optional)

4 eggs

4 cups mixed greens or arugula (optional)

2 plum tomatoes, cut into wedges and salted

3 radishes, thinly sliced (optional)

½ cup tender artichoke hearts (optional)

a handful of pitted Niçoise, Kalamata, or other black olives

1. <u>Vinaigrette</u>: Combine the ingredients in a jar. Cover and shake well to emulsify. Set aside.

2. <u>Salmon</u>: Place the lemon, salt, pepper, and 1½ to 2-inches water into a straight-sided pan. Cover and bring the poaching liquid to a boil. Lower the heat and add the salmon. Cover and simmer for about 6 to 8 minutes or until opaque. Transfer to a clean plate and chill at least 10 minutes in the refrigerator.

3. <u>Blanch the green beans</u>: Prepare a container of ice water. This will be used to shock the green beans so they stay nice and green. Bring a pot of water to a boil. Drop in the green beans and boil 2-4 minutes. Remove (with tongs or mesh skimmer) and drop them into the ice bath. Remove when cool and set aside.

4. <u>Boil the eggs</u>: Bring the water back to a boil. Add the eggs. Boil 8 minutes for jammy eggs. Boil 10 minutes if you prefer firmer yolks. Then either plunge the eggs into the ice bath or run under cold tap water until cool. Roll the eggs on a hard surface with your palm to crush the eggshells. Peel under running water. Set aside.

5. <u>To assemble</u>: Gently mix the greens with just enough dressing to coat. Spread the greens onto a serving plate. Arrange the green beans, tomatoes, radishes, artichokes, and olives however you prefer. Flake chunks of salmon onto the salad. Cut the eggs in half and add to the salad. Spoon some of the dressing over the salmon.

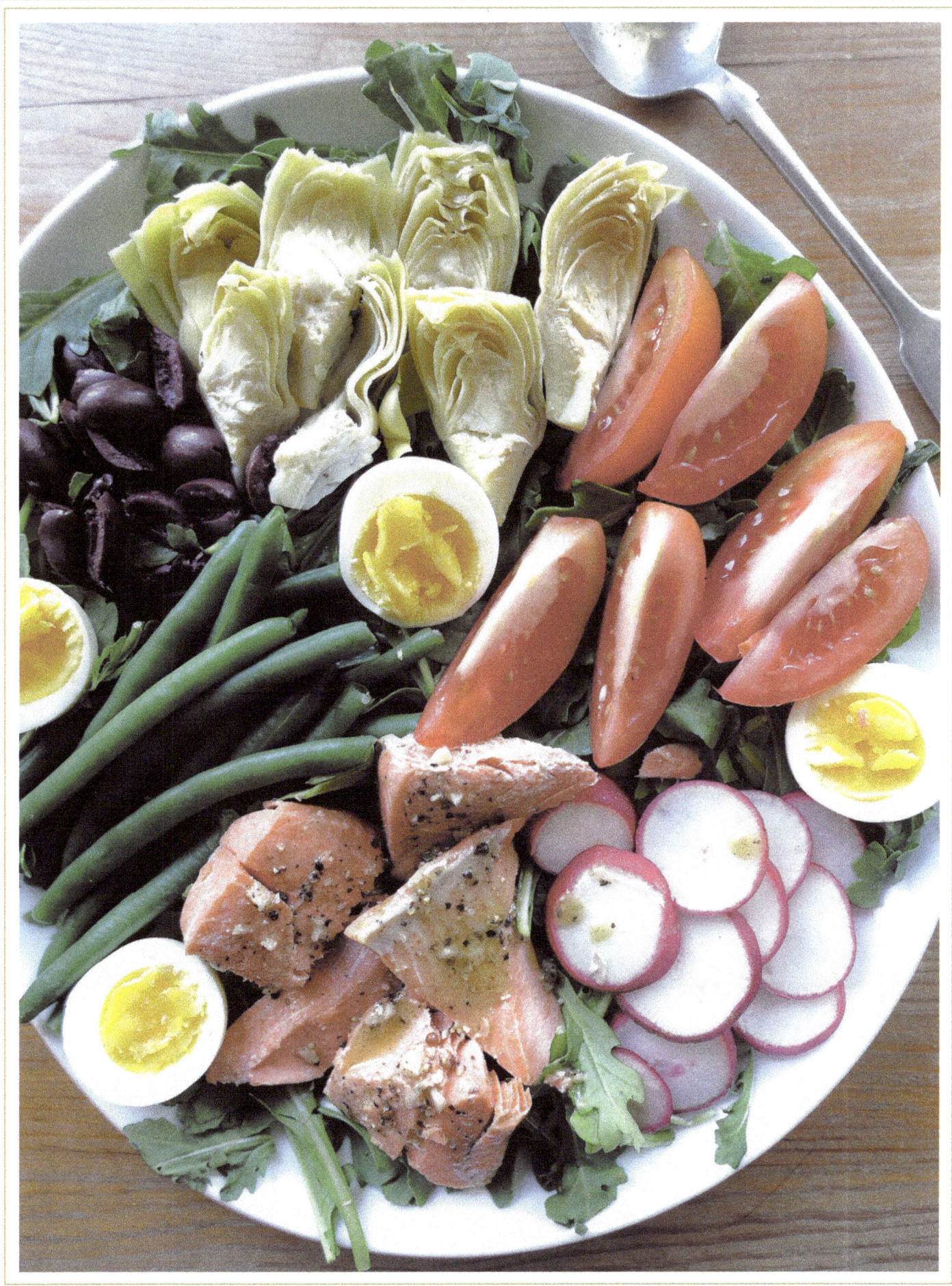

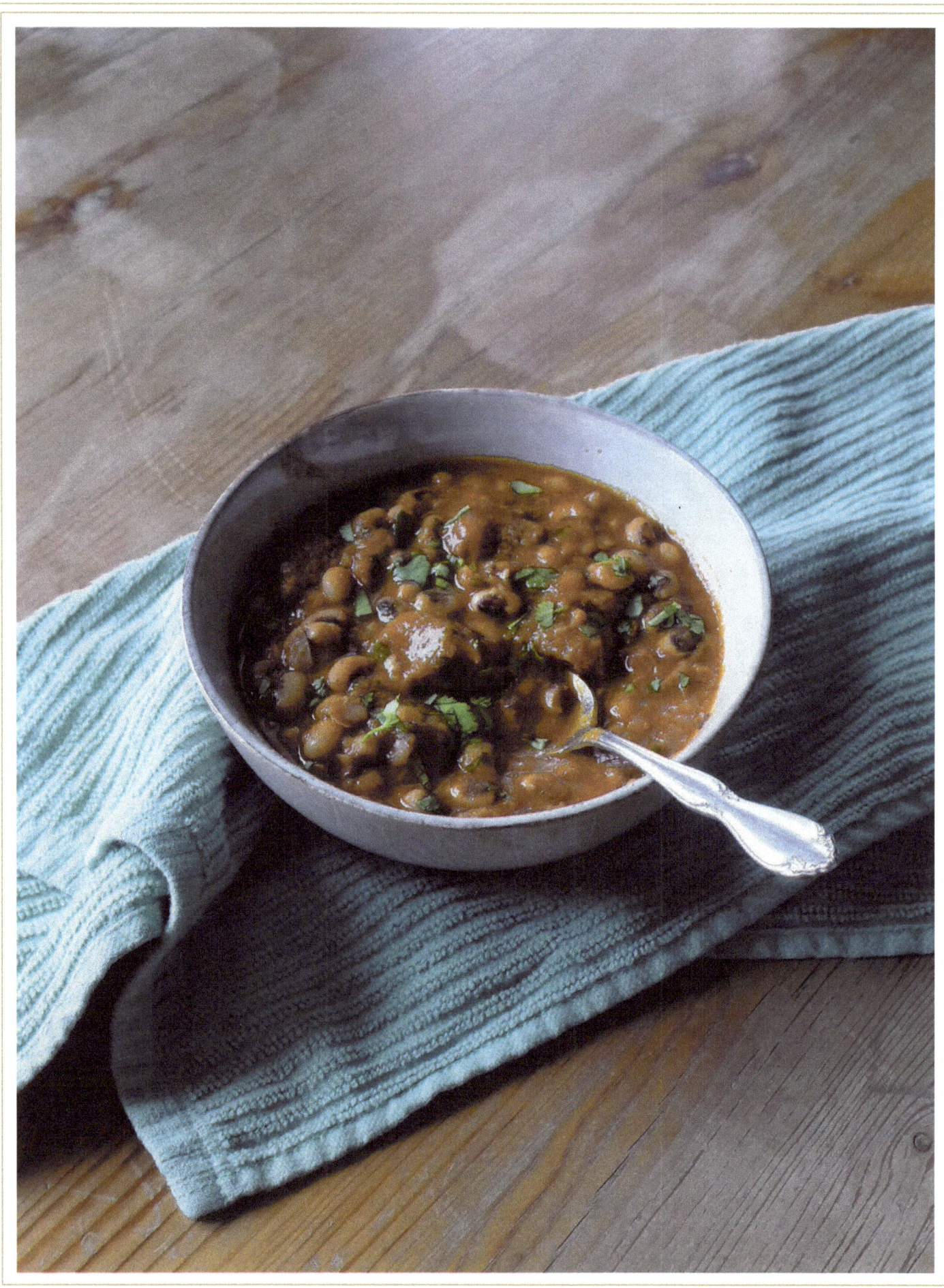

SOUPS

Lemon & Cilantro Lentil Soup

Red Lentil Soup with Dill Hot Sauce

Orange Soup with Fried Sage

Provençal Vegetable Soup with Herb Pistou

Greek Pork & Celery Stew

White Chicken Noodle Soup

Libyan Minted Lamb Soup

Egyptian Black-Eyed Pea Stew

Maltese Fish Soup

Salmon Pot

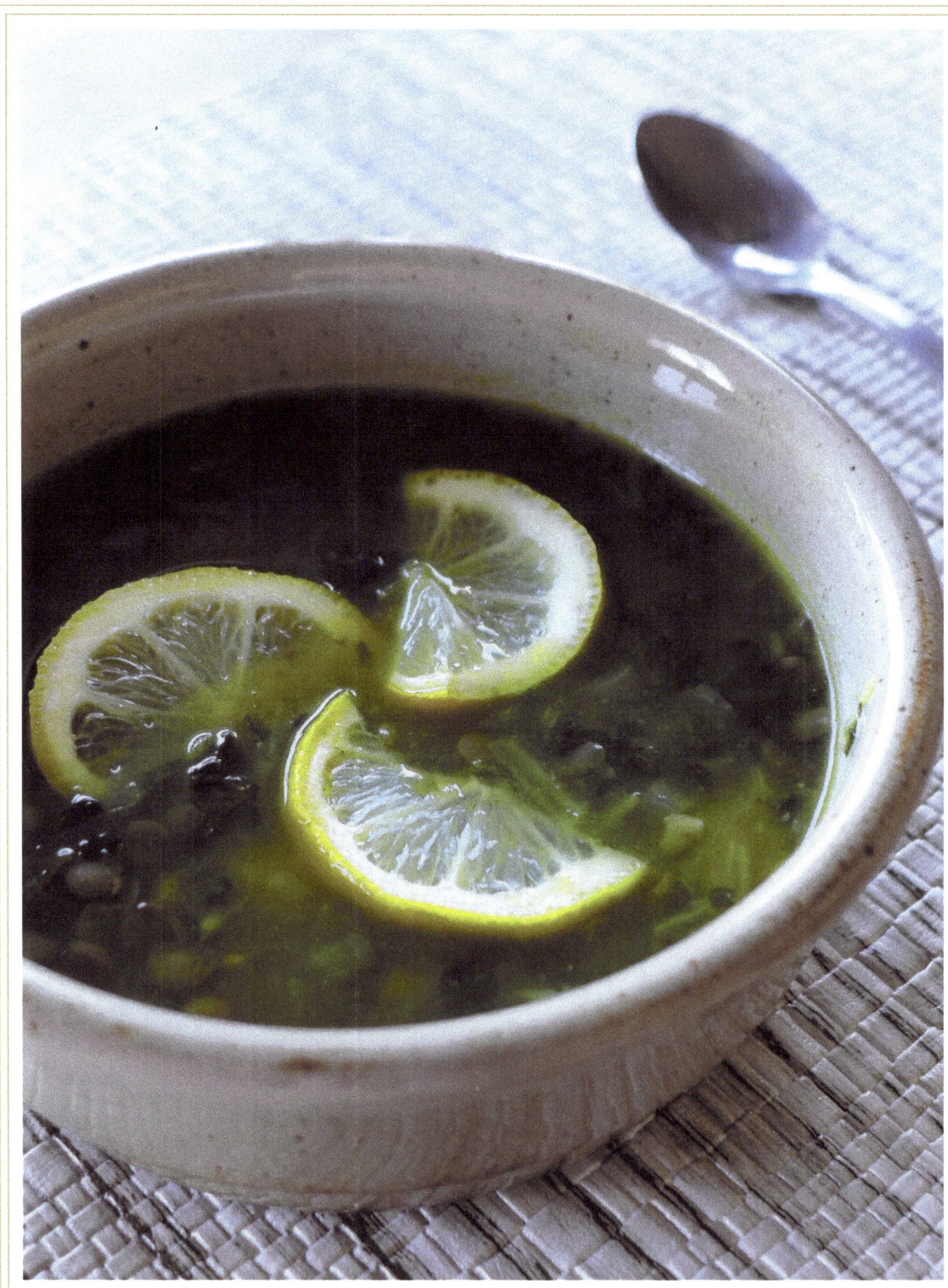

Lemon & Cilantro Lentil Soup

Cilantro and greens simmer with lentils to make this lemon-kissed Lebanese soup.

1 bunch cilantro, end trimmed
2 Tbsp. extra-virgin olive oil
1 onion, diced
1 Tbsp. minced garlic
1 bay leaf
1 cup brown lentils, inspected for pebbles and rinsed
6 cups water or lightly flavored stock/broth (vegetable or chicken)
½ tsp. sea salt
1 tsp. ground cumin
1 tsp. ground coriander
¼ tsp. turmeric
2 or 3 medium potatoes, peeled and roughly chopped
1 bunch Swiss chard or Tuscan kale (or a few handfuls of baby greens, spinach, or arugula), cleaned and chopped
fresh lemon juice, to taste (serve with additional lemon wedges)

1. Chop the entire bunch of cilantro in half. Chop the leafy end and reserve for later. Mince about ¼ cup of the stems and set aside (they're loaded with flavor).

2. Heat the oil, onions, garlic, bay leaf, and cilantro stems in a soup pot. Cook, stirring occasionally, until the onions are translucent.

3. Stir in the lentils. Add water or a lightly flavored stock. Bring to a boil, then reduce the heat. Cover and simmer for 20 minutes.

4. Discard the bay leaf. Add the salt, spices, potatoes, and cilantro leaves. Simmer for another 20 minutes.

5. Finally add the greens. Cook 5-10 minutes or until tender. Off the heat, add lemon juice to taste.

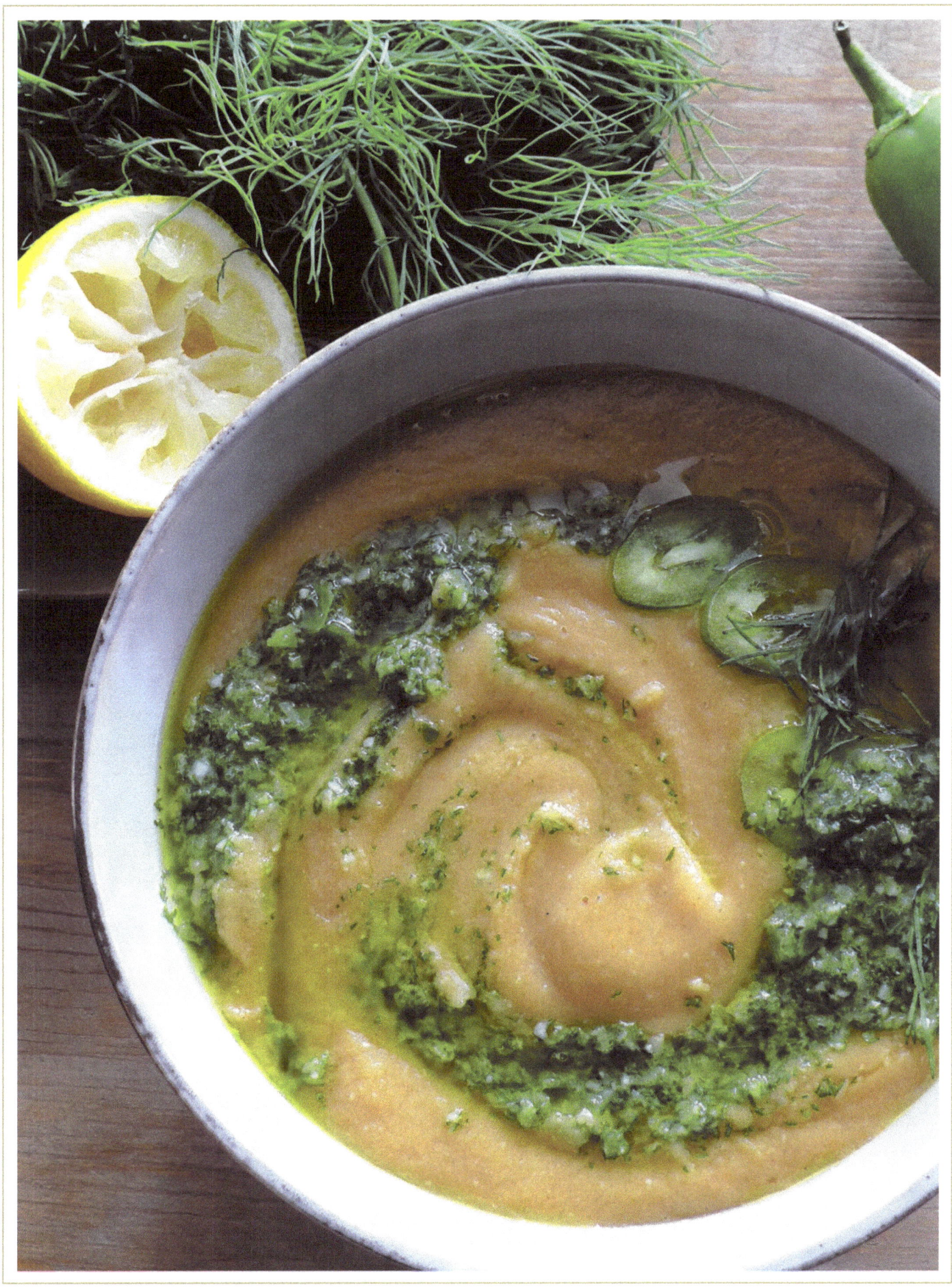

Red Lentil Soup with Dill Hot Sauce

Comforting and nourishing, red lentil soup is an eastern Mediterranean staple. Swirl in some dill hot sauce if you dare.

3 Tbsp. extra-virgin olive oil
1 onion, chopped
3 carrots, peeled and chopped
7 garlic cloves, minced
dash sea salt, plus more to taste
3 Tbsp. tomato paste
1 tsp. ground cumin
1 tsp. paprika
freshly ground black pepper, to taste
1 cup red lentils, inspected for pebbles and rinsed
1 quart (4 cups) low-sodium chicken or vegetable stock
2 cups water
fresh lemon juice, to taste

Dill Hot Sauce
¼ cup (about ½-oz.) fresh dill
1 to 2 jalapenos, cored and roughly chopped
3 garlic cloves, peeled
¼ cup extra-virgin olive oil
pinch sea salt

    1. Heat the oil in a soup pot. Add the onions, carrots, and garlic with a good dash of sea salt. Cook until the carrots are tender without browning the garlic.
    2. Stir in the tomato paste, spices, and lentils. Cook for a few minutes, then pour in the stock and water.
    3. Bring to a boil, then reduce the heat to low. Cover and gently simmer for 40 minutes or until the lentils are mushy. Stir occasionally.
    4. Purée with an immersion blender. If using a countertop blender, carefully blend in small batches, securing the lid. Season to taste with salt, pepper, and lemon.
    5. For the sauce: Process in a small food processor until smooth. Try a scoop in your next bowl of soup. It's great on fish, eggs, and dips too!

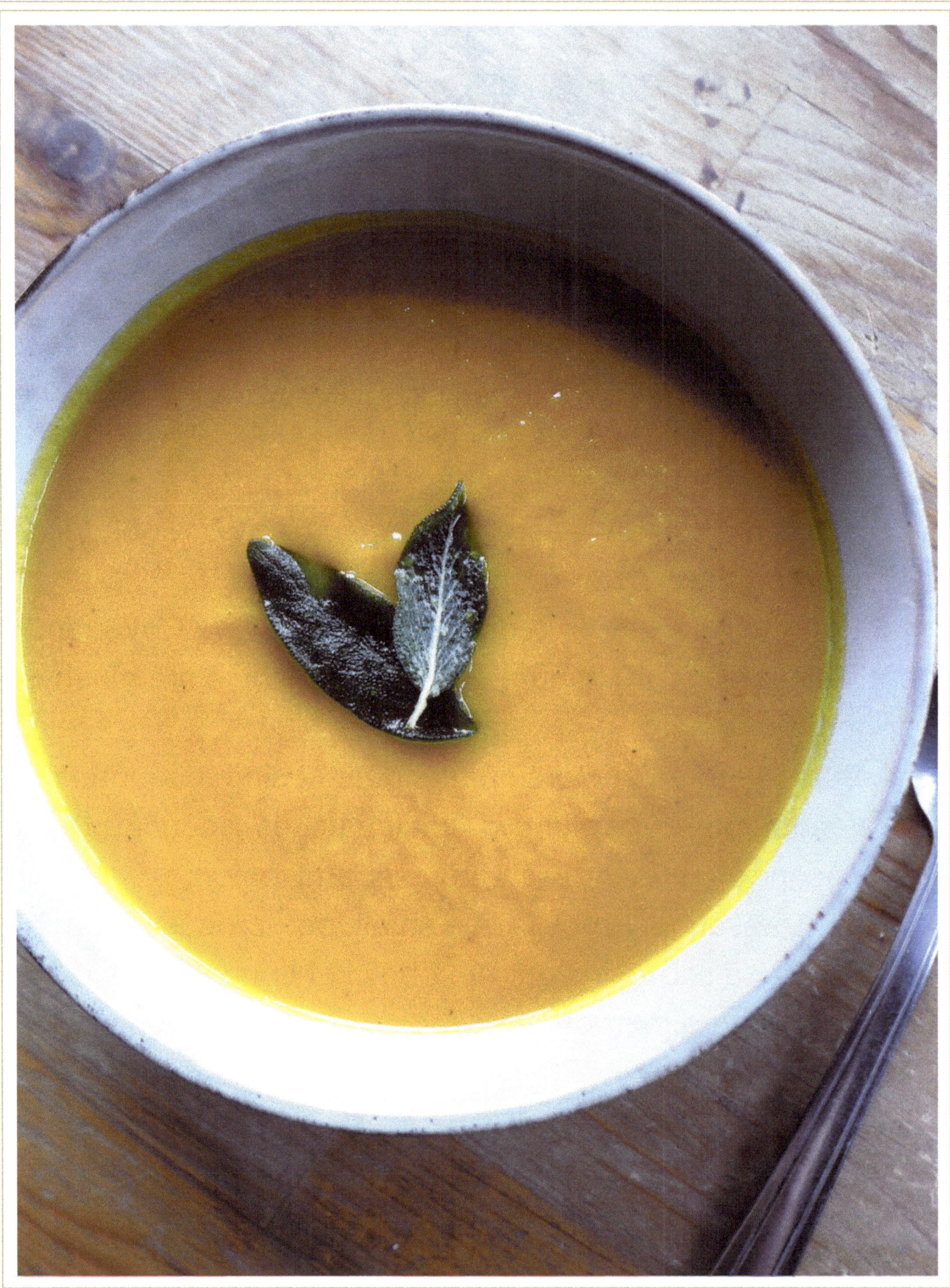

Orange Soup with Fried Sage

3 Tbsp. extra-virgin olive oil
8 whole sage leaves (for garnish)
sea salt
1 yellow onion, chopped
2 garlic cloves, minced
2 tsp. chopped fresh sage (½ tsp. rubbed sage)
freshly ground black pepper, to taste
1 lb. carrots, peeled and chopped
3 cups peeled and diced sweet potatoes, butternut squash, or pumpkin (or 10-oz. frozen diced sweet potatoes)
2 tsp. honey
low-sodium chicken or vegetable stock, to cover
pinch nutmeg

    1. Heat the oil in a soup pot over medium-high heat. Fry the sage leaves for just a few seconds until crisp—without browning. Carefully transfer to a plate lined with paper towel. Immediately sprinkle with sea salt. Set aside.

    2. Add the onions, garlic, chopped sage, salt, and pepper to the pot. Cook until the onions are soft, without browning the garlic.

3. Stir in the carrots, sweet potatoes, and honey. Add enough stock to cover by an inch. Bring to a boil, then reduce the heat to low. Cover and simmer for 25 minutes or until the vegetables are mushy. Stir occasionally.

4. Freshly grate nutmeg into the pot. Purée with an immersion blender or counter-top blender. Season to taste with salt and pepper. Garnish bowls with fried sage leaves.

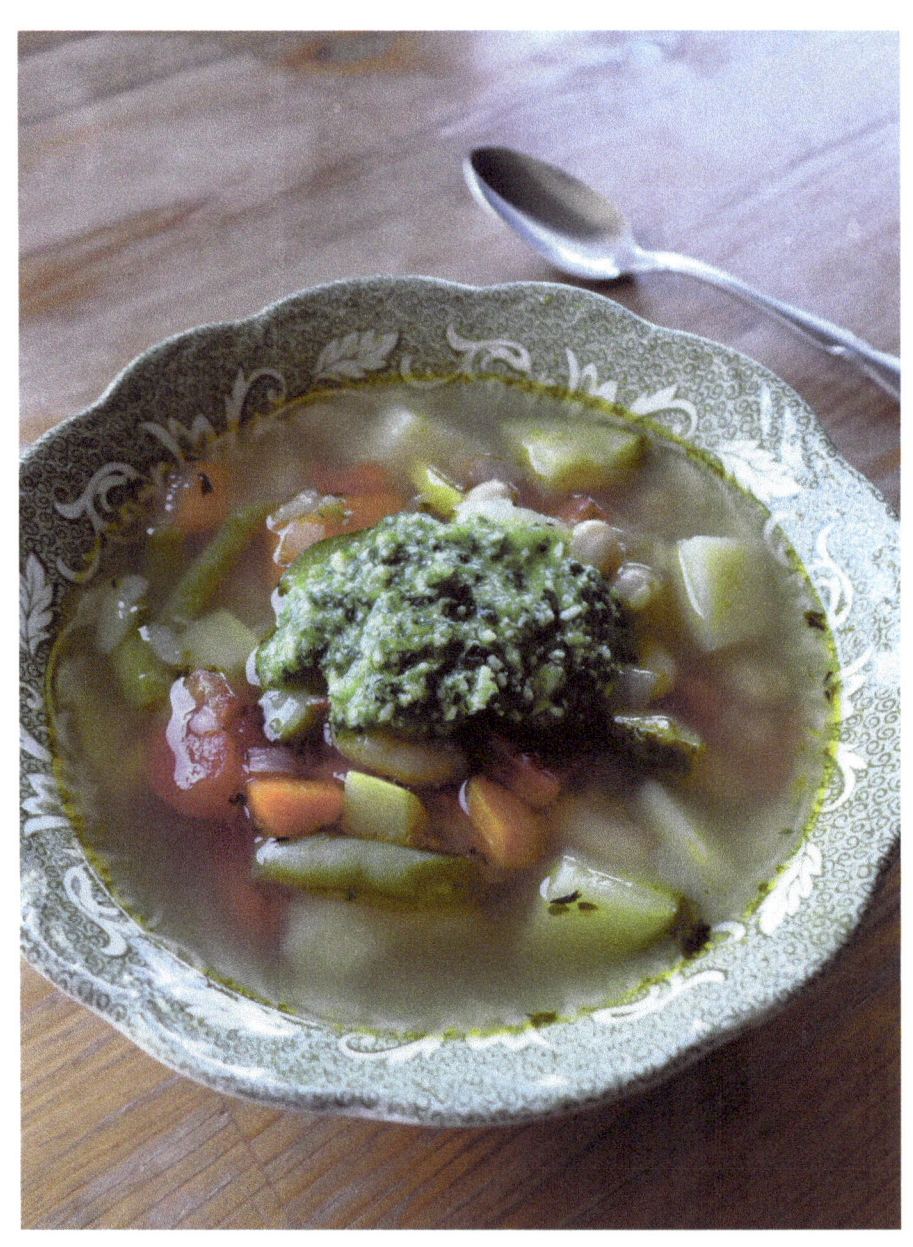

Provençal Vegetable Soup with Herb Pistou

Lunch like you're on the French Riviera with this summer vegetable soup. A swirl of fresh pistou infuses the simple broth with bright herbaceous flavor.

Herb Pistou (substitute: pesto)
½ cup (packed) basil leaves
¼ cup roughly chopped flat-leaf parsley
¼ cup roughly chopped scallions
¼ cup freshly grated parmesan cheese
2 Tbsp. extra-virgin olive oil
1 Tbsp. lemon juice, or more to taste
1 garlic clove, peeled
pinch sea salt

Vegetable Soup
2 Tbsp. extra-virgin olive oil
1 large onion, diced
2 carrots, chopped
2 garlic cloves, minced
1 tsp. sea salt, or more to taste
freshly ground black pepper, to taste
2 bay leaves

1 medium zucchini, diced

1 yellow squash, diced

1 (14.5-oz.) fire-roasted diced tomatoes

2 potatoes, peeled and diced

a handful of green beans, cut into bite-sized pieces (about 1 cup)

1 (15-oz.) can cannellini beans, drained and rinsed

6 cups low-sodium chicken or vegetable stock

1. <u>To make pistou</u>: Process until smooth with a small food processor (or pound with a mortar and pestle). Reserve.

2. <u>For the soup</u>: Heat the oil in a large soup pot. Add the onions, carrots, garlic, salt, pepper, and bay leaves. Cook until the onions are translucent, stirring occasionally.

3. Stir in the zucchini, squash, tomatoes, potatoes, green beans, cannellini beans, and stock. Simmer for 25 minutes. Add salt to taste.

4. Remove from the heat. Just before serving, stir in half of the pistou. Serve the rest on the side. Top with additional parmesan.

Greek Pork & Celery Stew

This cold weather stew pairs celery leaves with lean pork.

3 Tbsp. extra-virgin olive oil
1 lb. pork tenderloin, diced large (remove silver skin)
sea salt and black pepper, to taste
1 yellow onion, diced
1 cup chopped celery leaves (Seek the leafiest stalk you can find)
4 scallions, sliced
3 garlic cloves, minced
1 tsp. dried oregano
1 bay leaf
1 (15-oz.) can white beans, drained and rinsed (optional)
1 bunch Tuscan Kale, cleaned and chopped (optional)
1 quart (4 cups) low-sodium chicken or vegetable stock
water (to cover)
2 Tbsp. chopped fresh dill

Avgolemono
2 whole eggs (room temperature)
1 lemon, juiced
plus 1 cup of the soup broth to temper

1. Heat the oil in a soup pot over medium-high heat. Season the pork with salt and pepper to taste, then brown on all sides.

2. Add the onions, celery, and scallions, with a pinch of sea salt. Cook over medium heat until the onions are translucent, stirring occasionally. Stir in the garlic, oregano, and bay leaf. Cook for another minute.

3. Add the beans and kale if using, stock, and enough water to cover by an inch. Bring to a boil, then reduce the heat to low. Cover and simmer for 40 minutes or until the pork is very tender. Discard the bay leaf. Stir in the fresh dill.

4. <u>Finish with avgolemono</u>: Whisk together the eggs and lemon juice in a bowl. Whisk a cup of warm soup broth into the mixture. Pour it into the soup and stir well. Gently cook for another 2 minutes. Do not boil because the eggs may curdle. Season with salt and pepper. Serve with crusty bread.

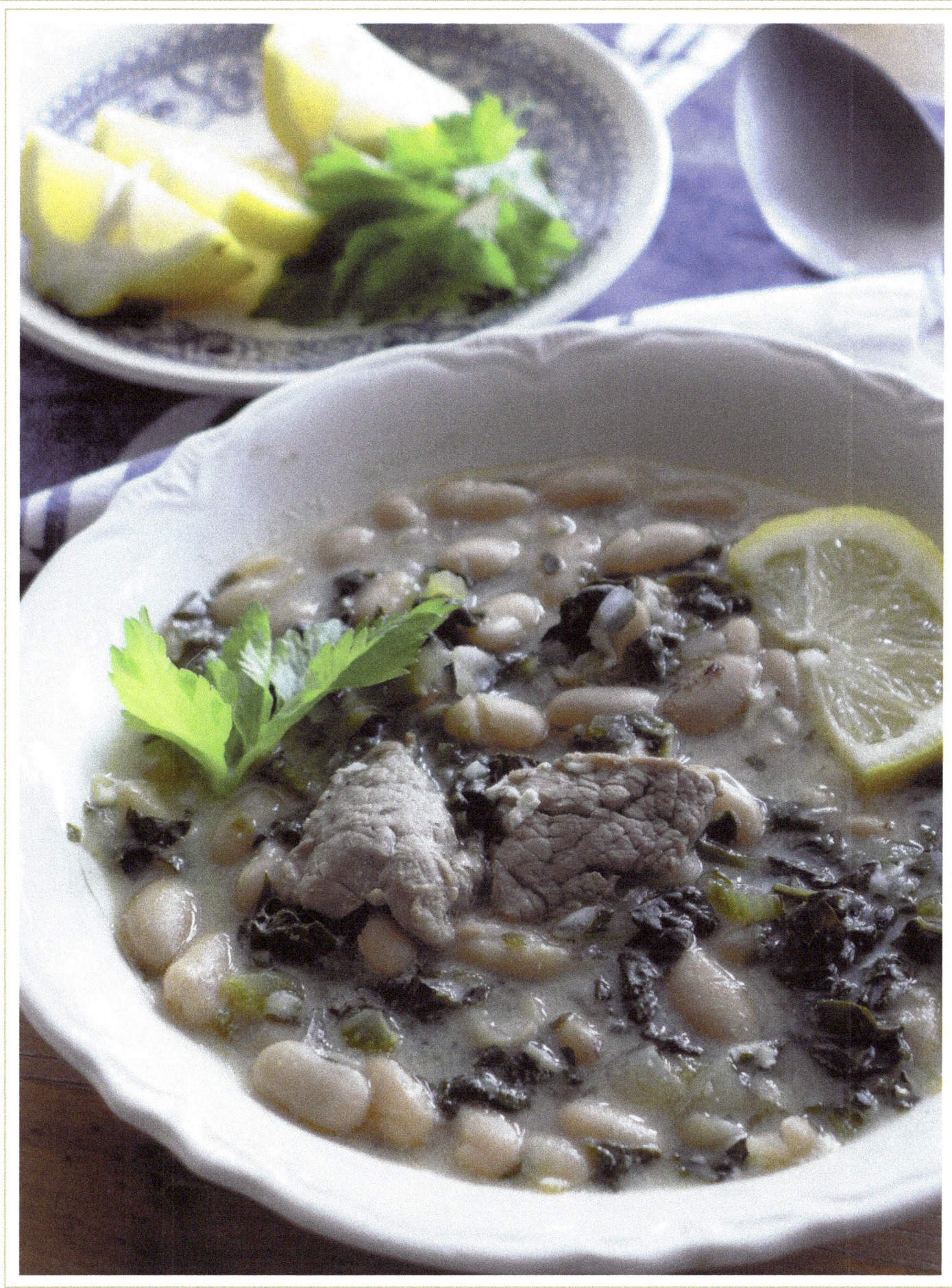

White Chicken Noodle Soup

A whisper of cinnamon perfumes this North African chicken noodle soup.

2 Tbsp. extra-virgin olive oil
3 chicken thighs or 4 drumsticks, skin removed (or combination of parts)
1 yellow onion, diced
1 cinnamon stick (or ½ tsp. ground cinnamon)
1 bay leaf
sea salt and freshly ground black pepper, to taste
1 (15-oz.) can chickpeas, drained and rinsed
1 quart (4 cups) low-sodium chicken stock
2 cups water
1 cup broken vermicelli or angel-hair pasta

El-Akda
1 egg yolk
1 lemon, juiced
2 Tbsp. chopped fresh parsley
plus 1 cup of the soup broth to temper

1. Heat the oil in a soup pot and add the chicken, onions, cinnamon, bay leaf, salt, and pepper. Cook over medium heat until the onions are translucent.

2. Add the chickpeas, chicken stock, and water. Bring to a boil, then reduce the heat to low. Cover and simmer for 30 minutes.

3. Transfer the chicken to a clean plate. Pick the meat off the bones when cool enough to handle. Add the chicken meat and pasta to the pot. Simmer for another 5 minutes.

4. <u>To finish</u>: Whisk together the egg yolk, lemon juice, and parsley in a bowl. Whisk a cup of soup broth into the mixture. Pour it into the soup and stir well. Gently cook for another 2 minutes. Season with salt and pepper.

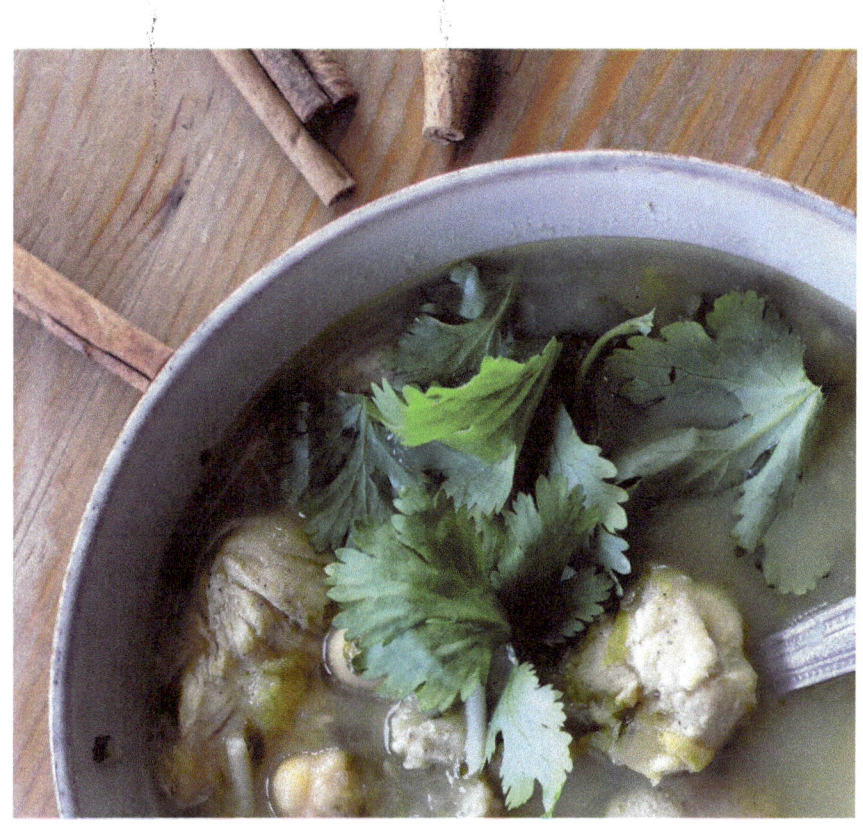

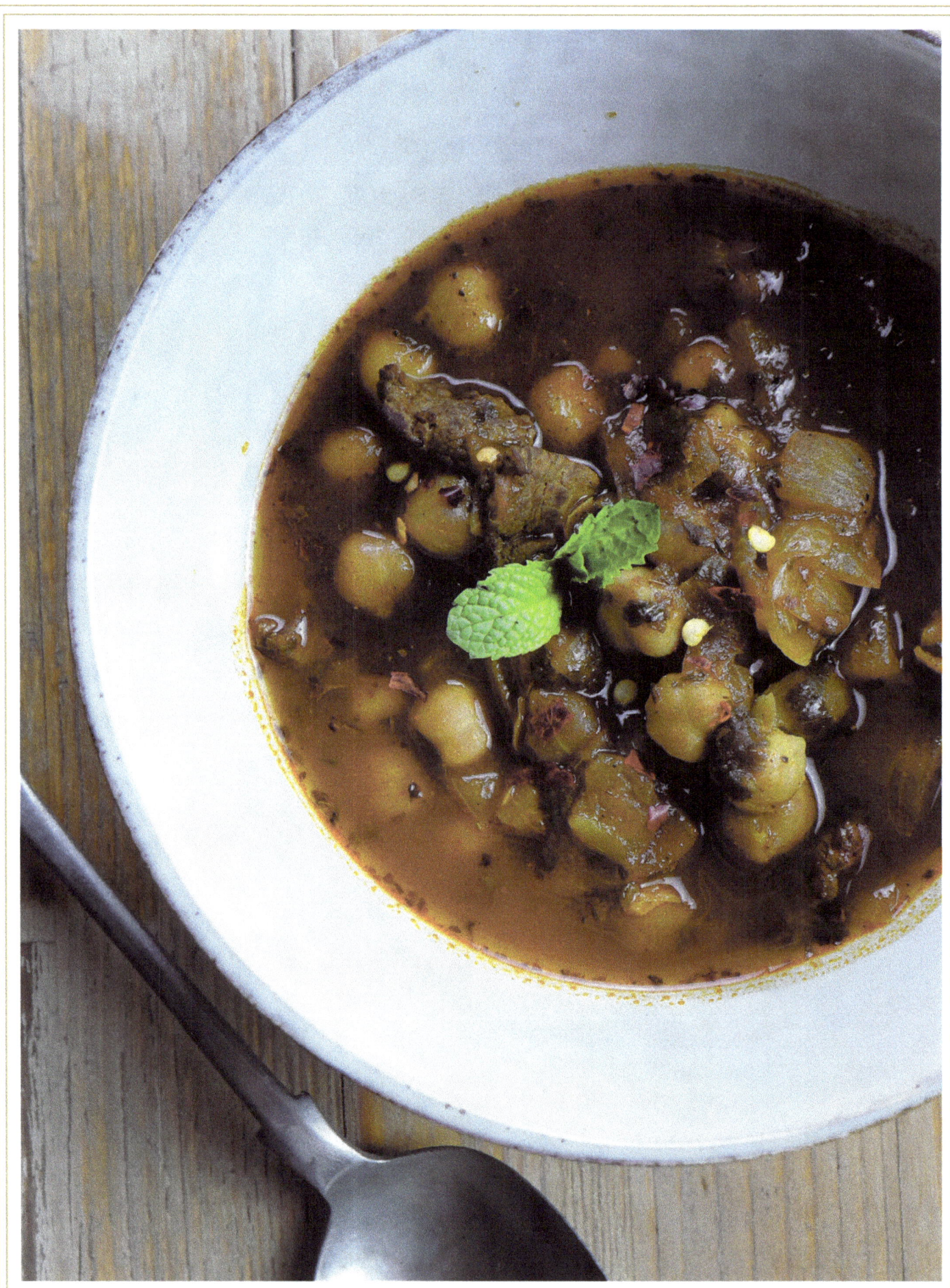

Libyan Minted Lamb Soup

This restorative red soup is flavored with warming spices, fresh green herbs, and hand-crushed spearmint.

2 Tbsp. extra-virgin olive oil
½ to 1 lb. boneless lamb meat, diced small (substitute: lean beef or chicken)
1 yellow onion, diced
dash sea salt, more to taste
3 garlic cloves, minced
3 Tbsp. tomato paste
½ tsp. turmeric
½ tsp. cinnamon
¼ tsp. cayenne pepper
freshly ground black pepper, to taste
½ cup chopped parsley, divided
½ cup chopped cilantro, divided
1 (15.5-oz.) can chickpeas, drained and rinsed
1 (14.5-oz.) can diced tomatoes
1 quart (4 cups) chicken or vegetable stock
2 cups water
1 Tbsp. dried mint (plus more to garnish)
fresh lemon juice, to taste

1. Heat the oil in a soup pot. Add the lamb, onions, and sea salt. Cook over medium heat until the onions are translucent.

2. Stir in the garlic, tomato paste, spices, and half of the fresh herbs. Cook for a few minutes without browning the garlic.

3. Pour in the chickpeas, tomatoes, stock, and water. Stir well. Bring to a boil. Then reduce the heat to low and cover. Simmer for 25 minutes.

4. Stir in the rest of the fresh herbs. Rub the dried mint between your hands and drop it into the soup. Add more sea salt and lemon if needed.

5. Ladle soup into bowls and sprinkle with additional dried mint. Serve with crusty bread.

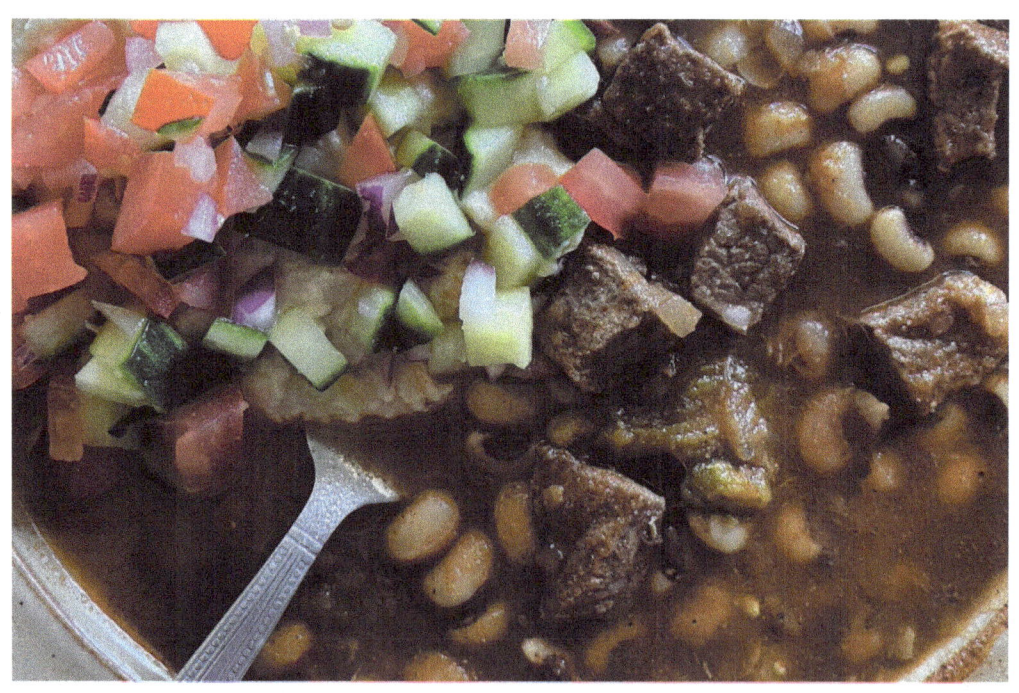

Egyptian Black-Eyed Pea Stew

This hearty stew features iron-rich lean beef and black-eyed peas. Just omit the beef and use vegetable stock for a new plant-based favorite.

2 cups (1 lb.) dried black-eyed peas
water (to boil)
2 Tbsp. extra-virgin olive oil
½ to 1 lb. boneless lean beef, diced (Chuck, round, sirloin and tenderloin are lean cuts.)
1 yellow onion, diced
1 tsp. sea salt, or more to taste
1 green chili pepper, minced (or toss in the whole pepper)
1 Tbsp. minced garlic
1½ tsp. ground cumin
1 tsp. ground coriander
¼ tsp. cinnamon
freshly ground black pepper, to taste
1 (6-oz.) can tomato paste
1 quart (4 cups) beef or vegetable stock
2 cups water
chopped cilantro or parsley (to garnish)
accompaniments: crusty bread or rice

1. <u>For the black-eyed peas</u>: Soak overnight in water. Drain and rinse. Boil in fresh water for 30 minutes or until tender. Drain and set aside.

2. <u>For the stew</u>: Heat the olive oil in a soup pot. Brown the beef if using. Stir in the onions and salt. Cook until the onions are translucent.

3. Add the green pepper, garlic, spices, and tomato paste. Cook for a few minutes without browning the garlic.

4. Stir in the cooked black-eyed peas, stock, and water. Bring to a boil, then reduce the heat to low. Cover and gently simmer for 45 minutes. Stir occasionally and add water if needed.

5. Ladle the stew into bowls and sprinkle with chopped herbs. Serve with crusty bread or ladle over rice instead.

Maltese Fish Soup

1 cup cooked brown rice
2 Tbsp. extra-virgin olive oil
1 yellow onion, diced
1 Tbsp. minced garlic (heaping)
sea salt
1 Tbsp. tomato paste

1 tsp. dried marjoram
freshly ground black pepper
1 bay leaf
1 (14.5-oz.) can diced tomatoes
1 quart (4 cups) vegetable or fish stock
1 cup water
1 lb. (about 3) white fish fillets (Cod, haddock, pollock, halibut, etc. Frozen is fine.)
1 Tbsp. chopped parsley
1 Tbsp. chopped mint (optional)
1 lemon, cut into wedges

1. Prepare the rice: Cook according to the directions on the package. Use up leftover rice if you have it. Set aside.
2. Sauté the onions and garlic in the oil with a pinch of salt until soft. Add the tomato paste, marjoram, pepper, and bay leaf. Cook for a minute.
3. Stir in the tomatoes, stock, and water. Bring to a boil, then reduce the heat to a gentle simmer.
4. Poach fillets 5-10 minutes in the broth, then transfer to a clean plate. Flake into bite-sized pieces. Discard any bones.
5. Finally, add the fish and brown rice to the pot. Simmer for 5 minutes. Stir in the parsley and mint. Season to taste with lemon, salt, and pepper.

Salmon Pot

Here is a rustic stew created by Basque fishermen out at sea.

4 medium potatoes, peeled
1 Tbsp. extra-virgin olive oil
1 yellow onion, diced
1 green or red bell pepper, diced (or half of each)
2 garlic cloves, minced
sea salt
½ tsp. smoked paprika
⅛ tsp. cayenne pepper
1 bay leaf
1 quart (4 cups) vegetable or fish stock
1 lb. skinless salmon, cut into cubes and lightly seasoned with sea salt
crusty bread (accompaniment)

1. <u>Break the potatoes</u>: Instead of cutting, the authentic Basque technique is to break off chunks with a knife. The potato starch adds body to the broth.

2. <u>For the soup</u>: Heat the oil in a pot. Sauté onions, bell peppers, and garlic, with a dash of sea salt, until soft.

3. Add potatoes, paprika, cayenne, bay leaf, and stock. If needed add enough water to cover by an inch. Simmer for 30 minutes.

4. Turn off the heat; add salmon; then cover the pot. Let the salmon cook by the heat of the broth alone for 5 minutes. Season to taste with sea salt. Smash some of the potatoes against the side of the pot for a thicker stew. Serve with crusty bread.

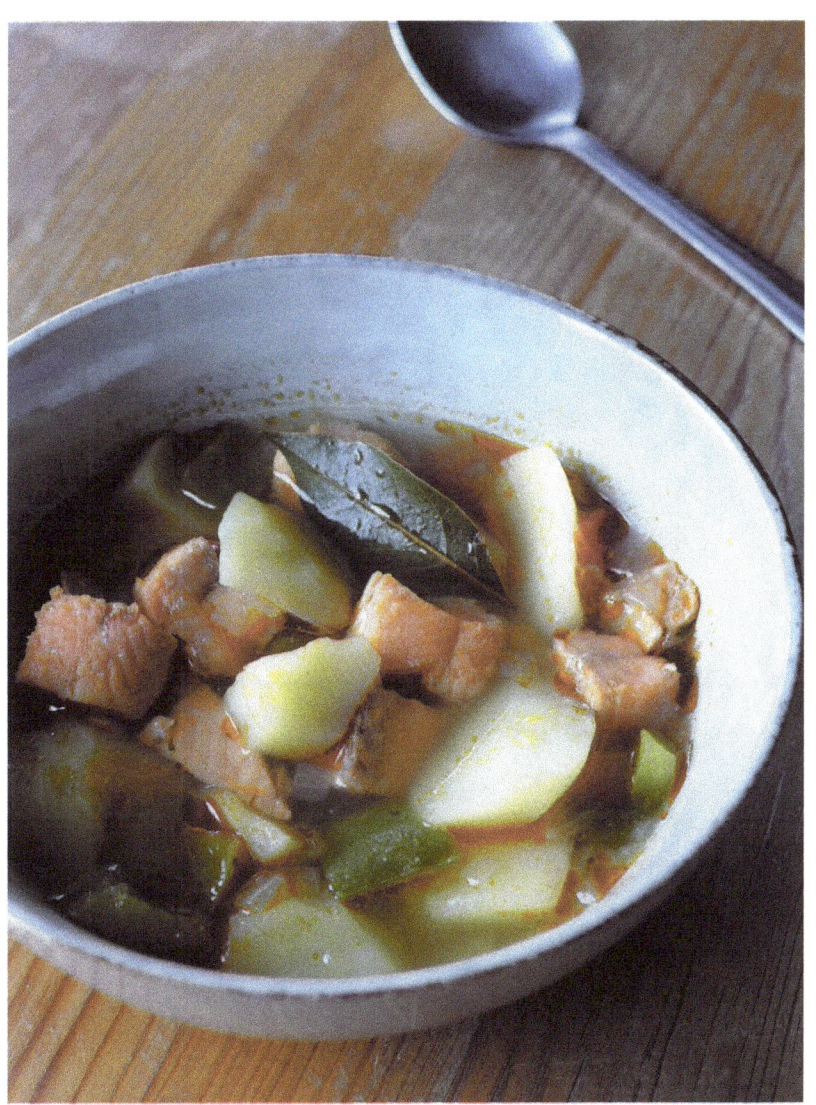

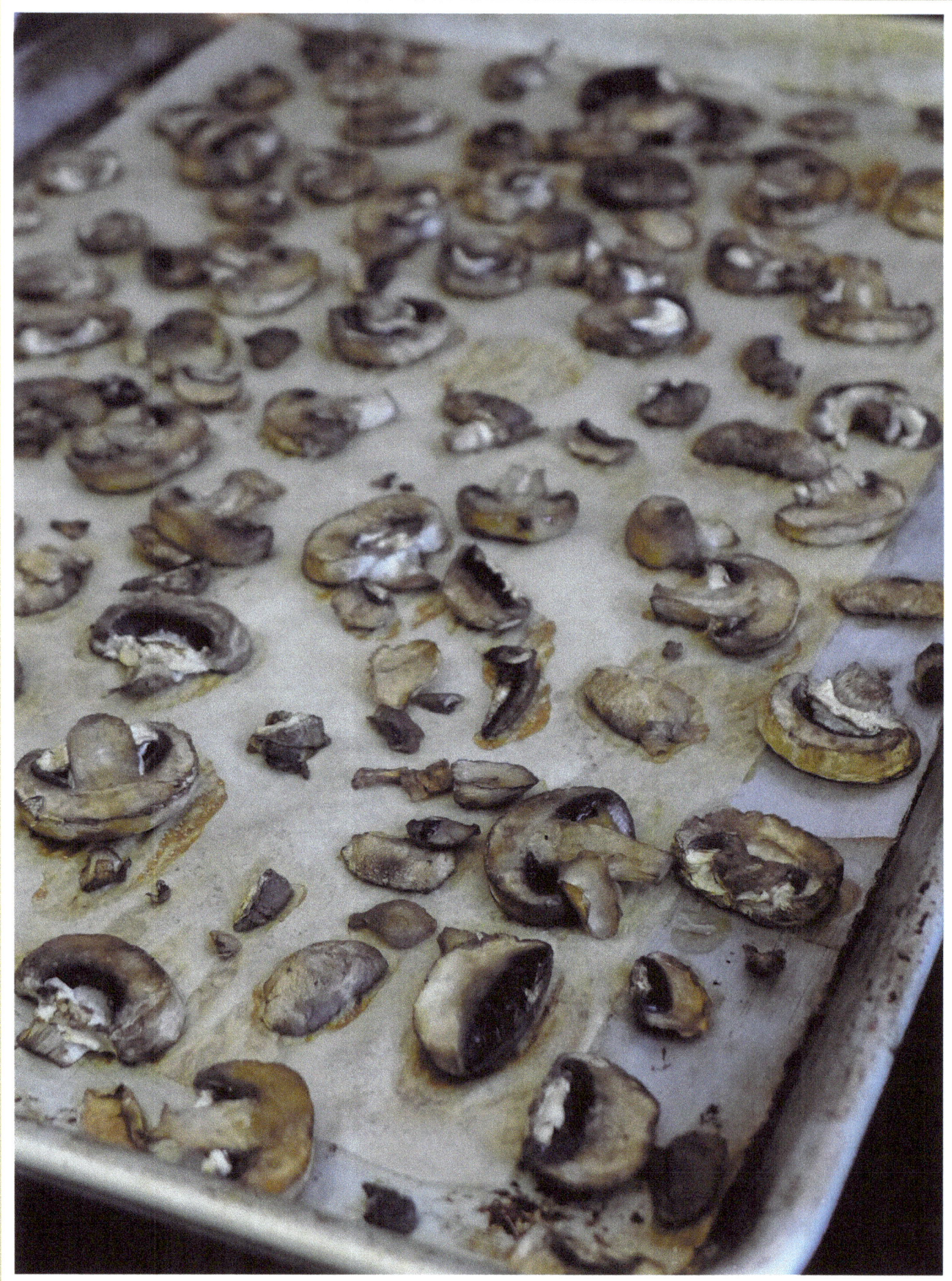

SIDES

Greek Dandelion Greens

Dalmatian Chard & Potatoes

Roasted Mushrooms Persillade

Roasted Brussels Sprouts

Balsamic Baby Broccoli

Stewed Sweet Peppers

Stewed Green Beans

Spinach Rice

Cilantro Rice

Yellow Rice Pilaf

Tomato Bulgur Pilaf

Mushroom Duxelles Brown Rice

Roasted Spaghetti Squash

Greek Dandelion Greens

Wild greens have been a household staple in Greece since ancient times.

2 bunches dandelion greens (or any greens)
2 Tbsp. good extra-virgin olive oil
1 lemon, juiced
sea salt and black pepper
crusty bread (to serve)

    1. Bring a pot of salted water to a boil. Coarsely chop and wash the greens. Boil until tender, then drain.
    2. Dress the greens with extra-virgin olive oil and lemon juice. Season with salt and pepper. Serve with a hunk of crusty bread.

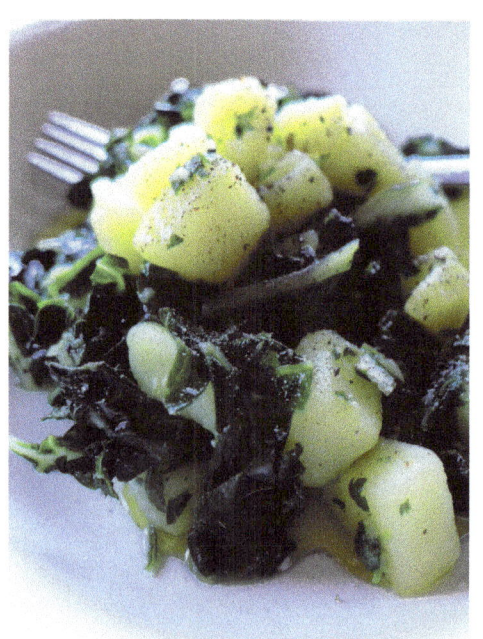

Dalmatian Chard & Potatoes

This garlicky Croatian dish is often paired with grilled fish, octopus, or squid from the Adriatic Sea.

2 bunches (approx. 2-lb.) Swiss chard (It will cook down to about 2 cups.)
4 medium potatoes, peeled and diced 1-inch
¼ cup extra-virgin olive oil
2 garlic cloves, minced
sea salt and black pepper

1. Bring a large pot of salted water to a boil.
2. Wash the Swiss chard to remove dirt. Tear off the leaves and coarsely chop. Set aside. Chop the stems too but keep separate.
3. Boil the stems and potatoes for 10 minutes. Now add the leaves and boil for another 5 minutes. Drain well.
4. Whisk together the olive oil and garlic. Pour over the potatoes and chard. Season with salt and pepper. Toss to combine. Leave the potatoes chunky or mash with some of the cooking liquid.

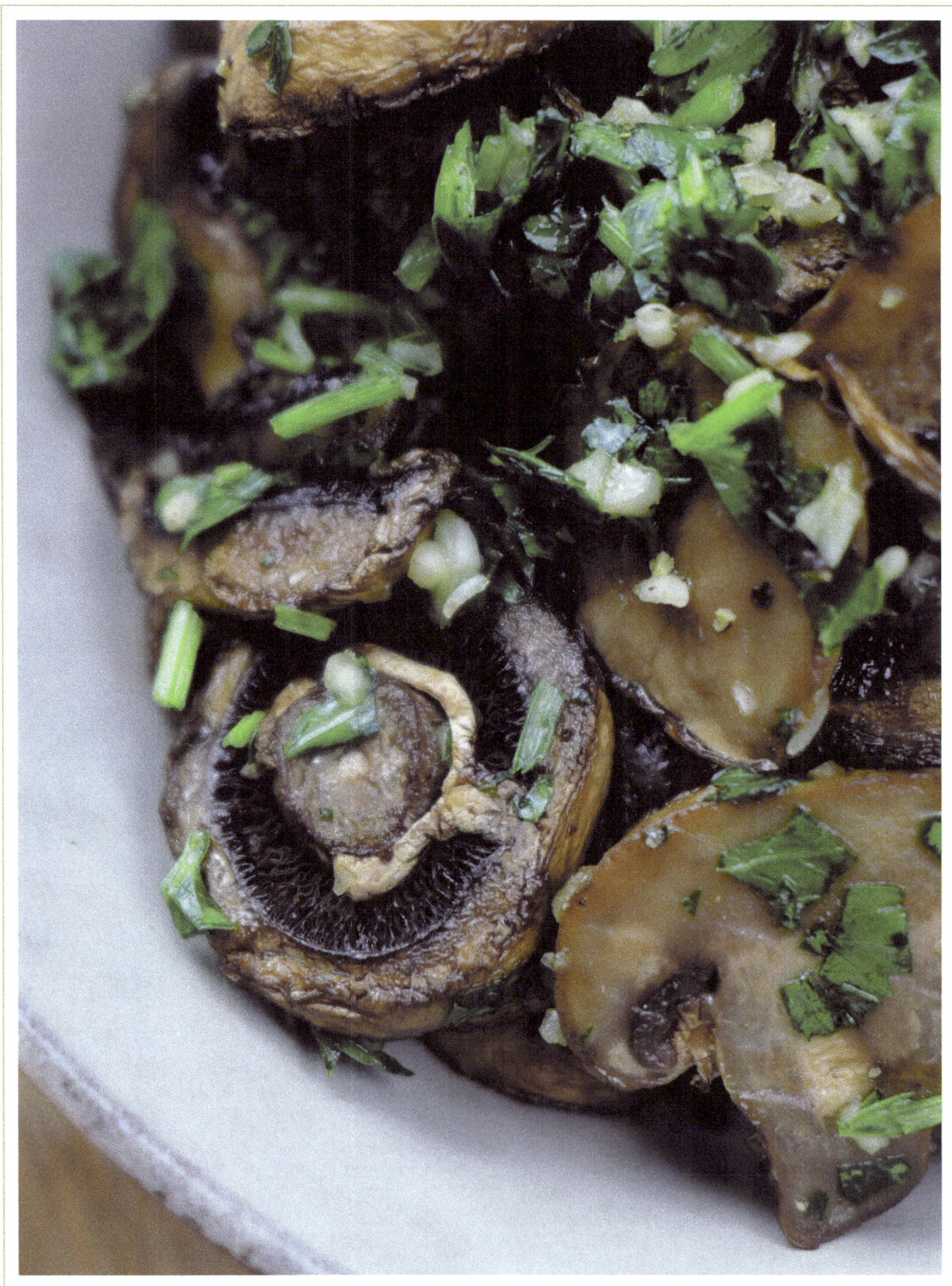

Roasted Mushrooms Persillade

1 lb. white or cremini mushrooms
extra-virgin olive oil
sea salt and freshly ground black pepper

Persillade
½ cup (packed) flat-leaf parsley leaves
3 Tbsp. extra-virgin olive oil
3 garlic cloves
pinch sea salt

1. Preheat your oven to 400°F. Wipe mushrooms clean with a damp paper towel just before roasting. Trim dark ends and cut larger mushrooms in half or quarters. Leave medium to small mushrooms whole.
2. Coat the mushrooms with a thin layer of olive oil. Season with salt and pepper. Space apart on a sheet pan. Roast for 20 minutes.
3. <u>For the persillade</u>: Finely mince by hand or use a small food processor.
4. Transfer the mushrooms to a large bowl and add the persillade. Mix well.

Roasted Brussels Sprouts

1 lb. Brussels sprouts
2 Tbsp. olive oil
2 Tbsp. red wine vinegar
½ tsp. granulated garlic
½ tsp. sea salt
¼ tsp. black pepper

1. Thinly shave off the brown ends. Then cut each sprout in half. Quarter larger ones.
2. Toss with the olive oil, vinegar, and seasonings. Arrange cut-side-down on a sheet pan.
3. Roast in an oven preheated to 425°F for 15-20 minutes or until fork-tender. After roasting, cut in half again if desired.

"Simple cuisine makes
the home great."
—Sardinian expression

Balsamic Baby Broccoli

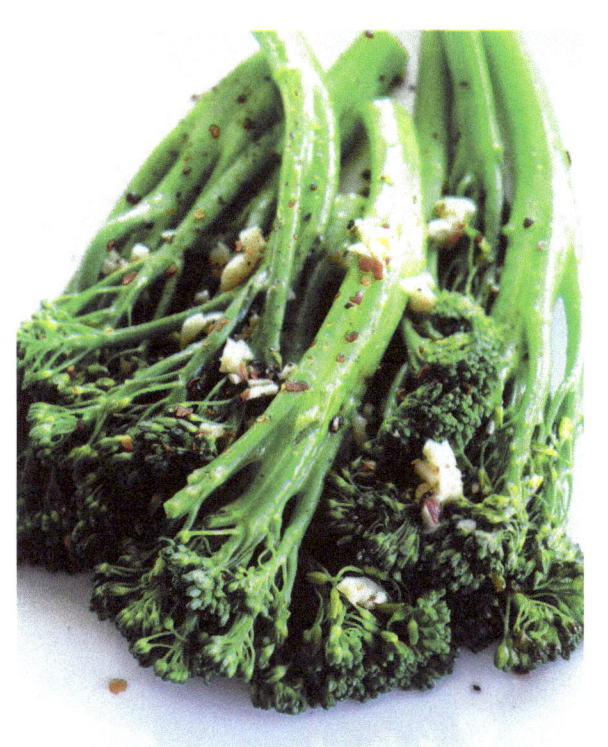

2 bunches baby broccoli,
　ends trimmed
　(substitute: broccoli florets)
2 Tbsp. extra-virgin olive oil
2 garlic cloves, finely minced
½ tsp. sea salt
1 Tbsp. balsamic vinegar

1. Bring a pot of water to a rolling boil. Add the broccoli and cook for 2 minutes. Drain well.

2. Heat the oil in a wide skillet over medium heat. Sauté the broccoli for about 3 minutes. Stir in the garlic; sprinkle with sea salt; and cook for another minute. Turn off the heat and drizzle the balsamic. Toss well.

Stewed Sweet Peppers

3 Tbsp. extra-virgin olive oil
1 onion, sliced
3 bell peppers, sliced (a combination of red, yellow, orange, or green)
½ tsp. sea salt
3 garlic cloves, sliced
1 tsp. paprika
pinch cayenne pepper
1 (28-oz.) can whole plum tomatoes, drained
½ cup water
chopped flat-leaf parsley or fresh basil (optional)

- Spoon these saucy peppers over pasta or polenta.
- Pair with grilled meat, fish, or scoop it with bread.
- Poach a few eggs into a freshly made batch.
- Toss with potatoes or rice.

1. Heat the oil in a wide pan. Add the onions and cook over medium heat until soft. Stir in the peppers and salt. Reduce the heat to low; cover; sweat the onions and peppers for 10 minutes, stirring occasionally.

2. Stir in the garlic, paprika, and cayenne.

3. Dump the tomatoes into a colander to drain. Crush them with clean hands. Add tomatoes and water to the pot. Mix well.

4. Cover and cook for another 15 minutes over low heat. Stir occasionally and add water as needed. Garnish with parsley or basil if desired.

Stewed Green Beans

Tomato stews are a mainstay of Mediterranean cooking – often based on green beans, legumes, okra, or peas.

¼ cup extra-virgin olive oil
1 large onion, chopped
2 garlic cloves, minced
1 Tbsp. tomato paste (heaping)
¼ tsp. sea salt, or more to taste
1 (15-oz.) can diced tomatoes
¼ cup chopped flat-leaf parsley
¼ tsp. cinnamon
¼ tsp. black pepper

2 or 3 medium potatoes, peeled and quartered
1 lb. green beans, trimmed
water
1 lemon, halved
accompaniments: crusty bread, feta

1. Heat olive oil in a large pot over medium heat. Cook the onions, garlic, tomato paste, and salt until the onions are translucent. Stir occasionally, mashing the tomato paste into the oil with your spoon.
2. Stir in the tomatoes, parsley, cinnamon, and pepper. Add the potatoes and green beans. Add enough water to cover. Bring to a boil, then reduce the heat to low. Cover and simmer for 30 minutes.
3. Remove the lid and simmer for another 15 minutes, or until the potatoes are fork-tender and some of the liquid has reduced.
4. Add salt and lemon juice to taste. Serve as a side or make it a meal with feta cheese and bread.

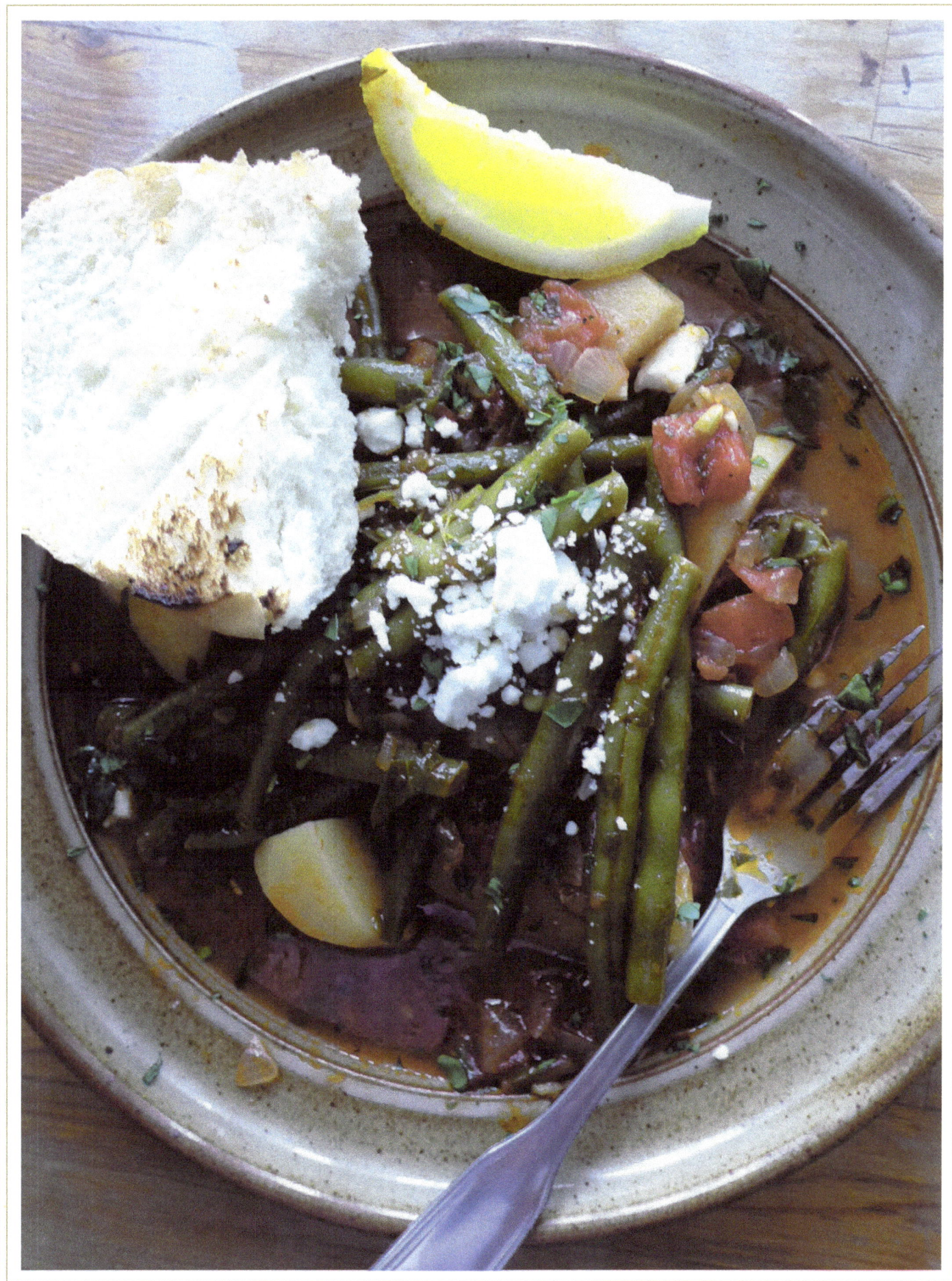

Spinach Rice

¼ cup extra-virgin olive oil
1 bunch scallions, sliced (or dice a medium onion)
2 Tbsp. tomato paste
1 lb. fresh spinach, washed (or use 10-oz. frozen spinach. Thaw and squeeze out as much water as you can.)
1 lemon, juiced
sea salt and freshly ground black pepper, to taste
1 Tbsp. chopped fresh dill (or 1 tsp. dried dill weed)
1 cup medium-grain rice, rinsed
2½ cups vegetable stock (or water)
feta cheese (to serve)
Pair with crusty bread or an olive oil fried egg

1. Heat oil in a large pot. Sauté scallions for a few minutes, then stir in tomato paste. Cook for another minute. Add the spinach in batches and cook until wilted.
2. Add lemon juice, salt, pepper, dill, rice, and stock. Bring to a boil, then reduce the heat to low. Cover and simmer for 20 minutes or until the rice is tender. Check occasionally and add water if needed. (This is more of a saucy rice dish as opposed to a fluffed one.)
3. Top with feta cheese and serve with crusty bread.

Cilantro Rice

Boiling rice in a big uncovered pot of water is liberating. And this method results in fluffy, separated grains every time.

6 cups water
1 bay leaf
1 tsp. sea salt
1 cup basmati rice (For brown rice cook according to package instructions.)
1 lime, juiced
½ lemon, juiced
2 Tbsp. extra-virgin olive oil
1 small bunch cilantro, chopped

1. Bring the water, bay leaf, and salt to a boil in a pot. Pour in the rice and boil uncovered for 12 minutes.
2. Dump the rice into a fine mesh strainer. Rinse with hot water. Place the strainer over a large bowl to drain for about 5 minutes.
3. Dump the rice into a large bowl and remove the bay leaf. Add citrus juice, olive oil, and cilantro. Season to taste with sea salt. Mix well.

Yellow Rice Pilaf

2 Tbsp. extra-virgin olive oil
½ cup diced onion
1 cup basmati rice, rinsed until water is clear
1¾ cups low-sodium chicken or vegetable stock
½ tsp. turmeric
½ tsp. ground cumin
¼ tsp. black pepper

1. Heat the oil in a pan. Add the onions and cook until translucent. Add the rice and sauté for a few minutes, stirring frequently.
2. Stir in the chicken stock and spices. Bring to a boil, then reduce the heat to low. Cover and simmer for 20 minutes or until tender. Turn off the heat and let the rice sit for 5 minutes. Fluff with a fork before serving.

Tomato Bulgur Pilaf

2 Tbsp. extra-virgin olive oil
1 yellow onion, diced
1 red bell pepper, diced (or green)
1 plum tomato, diced
sea salt
1 Tbsp. tomato paste
1 garlic clove, minced
½ tsp. paprika
½ tsp. smoked paprika
dash cayenne pepper
1 cup bulgur, rinsed (medium #2)
2 cups low-sodium chicken or vegetable stock

1. Heat the oil in a pot. Add the onions, peppers, tomatoes, and a good dash of sea salt. Cook until tender.
2. Stir in the tomato paste, garlic, paprika, smoked paprika, cayenne, and bulgur. Cook for two minutes.
3. Stir in the stock, then bring to a boil. Reduce the heat to low and immediately cover with a lid. Simmer for 12 minutes. Remove from heat and set aside for 10 minutes. Fluff with a fork before serving.

Mushroom Duxelles Brown Rice

2 Tbsp. extra-virgin olive oil

8-oz. cremini mushrooms, wiped clean with a damp paper towel and minced

¼ cup diced shallot or onion

2 garlic cloves, minced

1 Tbsp. chopped fresh thyme leaves (or 1 tsp. dried thyme)

1 bay leaf

dash sea salt

freshly ground black pepper, to taste

1 cup brown rice, rinsed

1 cup low-sodium chicken or vegetable stock

1 cup water

¼ cup chopped flat-leaf parsley

1. Heat the oil and add the mushrooms, onions, garlic, thyme, bay leaf, salt, and pepper. The salt will help draw moisture out of the mushrooms. Stir occasionally. Cook until the juices have evaporated leaving behind concentrated umami goodness.

2. Stir in the brown rice, stock, water, and parsley. Bring to a boil, then reduce the heat to low. Cover and cook for 45 minutes or until the liquid has evaporated.

Roasted Spaghetti Squash

1 spaghetti squash
1 Tbsp. extra-virgin olive oil
sea salt
freshly ground black pepper

1. Preheat your oven to 400°F. Cut the squash in half and scoop out the seeds. Rub the inside with olive oil and season with salt and pepper.
2. Place cut-side down on a parchment-lined sheet pan. Roast for 45 minutes or until fork-tender. Scrape out spaghetti-like strands of squash with a fork to serve.

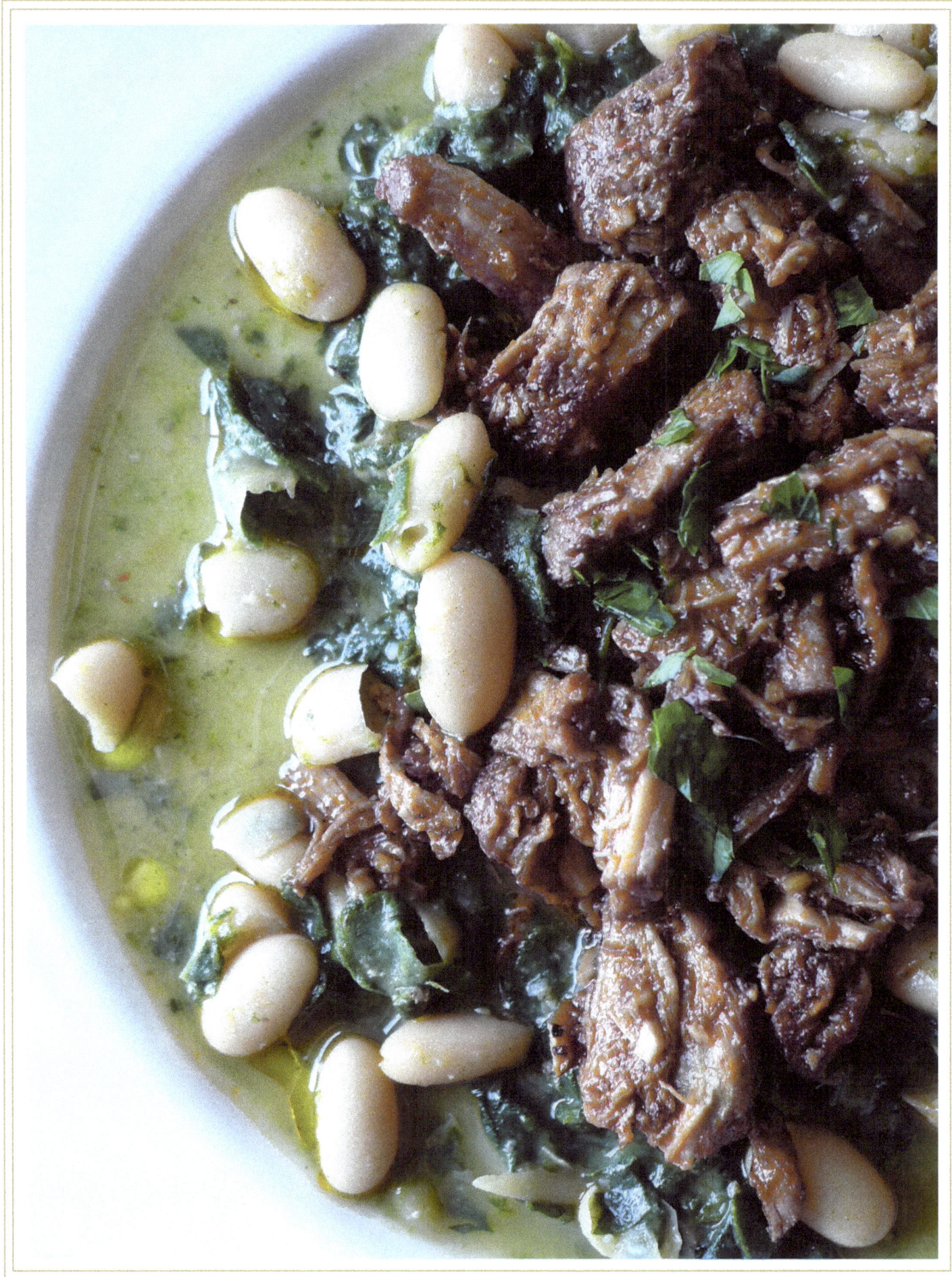

MAINS

Greek Vegetable Bake

Adriatic Herb Chicken

Egyptian Chicken with Sweet Potato Mash

Sultan's Apricot Chicken

Rosemary & Tomato Braised Chicken

Chianti Pulled Pork with Tuscan Kale

Salmoriglio Skillet Fish

Baked Chermoula Salmon

Parchment Baked Salmon
with Chive & Horseradish Sauce

Hvar Island Fish & Potatoes

Spicy Braised Fish

Spanish Garlic Shrimp

Greek Vegetable Bake

1 (15-oz.) can diced tomatoes
¼ cup extra-virgin olive oil
¼ cup flat-leaf parsley, chopped
3 garlic cloves, minced
2 tsp. dried oregano
1 tsp. dried mint (or 1 Tbsp. minced fresh spearmint)
1 tsp. sea salt
½ tsp. freshly ground black pepper

3 medium potatoes, peeled
1 or 2 bell peppers, any color
2 medium zucchini
1 medium eggplant
1 onion
1 lemon, halved (to finish)
accompaniments: brined feta cheese, crusty bread

    1. Preheat your oven to 375°F. Combine the tomatoes, olive oil, parsley, garlic, herbs, and spices in a 9×13-inch baking dish.
    2. Coarsely chop the vegetables and add to the baking dish. Mix well.

3. Roast uncovered for 90 minutes, stirring after about 45 minutes. Remove from the oven and finish with a generous squeeze of lemon. Serve with good feta cheese and sop up the juices with a hunk of crusty bread.

Adriatic Herb Chicken

Adriatic Herb Marinade
2 Tbsp. extra-virgin olive oil
1 tsp. lemon zest
¼ cup fresh lemon juice
1 Tbsp. chopped rosemary (1 tsp. dried rosemary)
1 Tbsp. chopped sage leaves (1 tsp. dried sage)
1 Tbsp. chopped thyme leaves (1 tsp. dried thyme)
2 garlic cloves, minced (or ½ tsp. granulated garlic)
1 tsp. sea salt
freshly ground black pepper, to taste
¼ tsp. ground nutmeg (optional)

1 lb. chicken thighs or skinless, boneless chicken breasts (pounded to an even thickness)

1. <u>Marinade</u>: Combine the marinade ingredients in a resealable plastic bag or container. Add the chicken and coat with the marinade. Marinate for at least an hour or overnight in the refrigerator.

2. Preheat your oven to 400°F. Line a rimmed sheet pan with parchment or use a 9×13-inch baking dish instead. Bring the chicken to room temperature on the counter just before cooking.

3. <u>Roast chicken thighs</u>: 35-40 minutes / boneless chicken breasts: 15-25 minutes
or until chicken reaches an internal temperature of 165°F at its thickest part. Cooking time will vary depending on the size and thickness of each piece. Rest for 10 minutes before cutting.

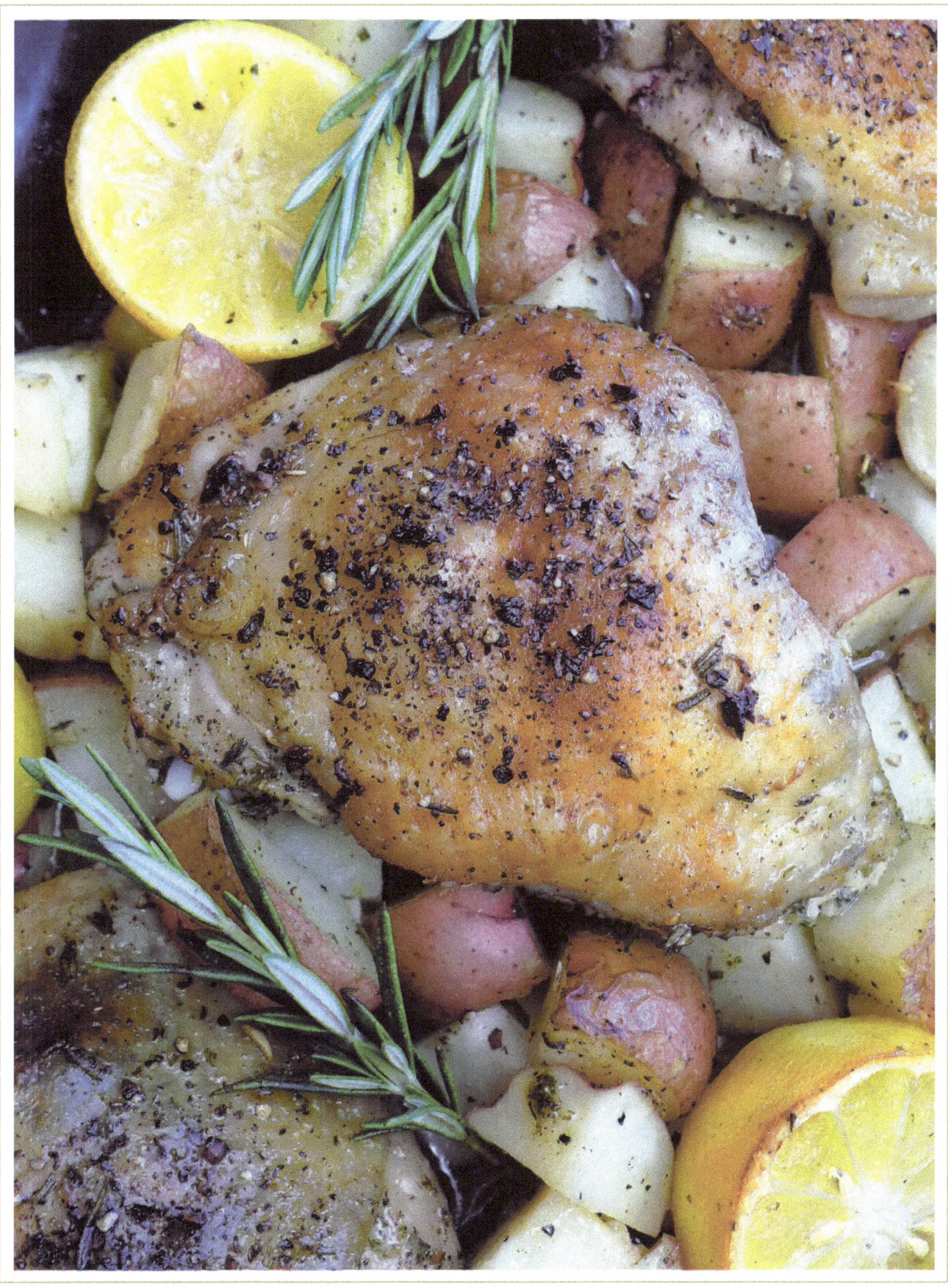

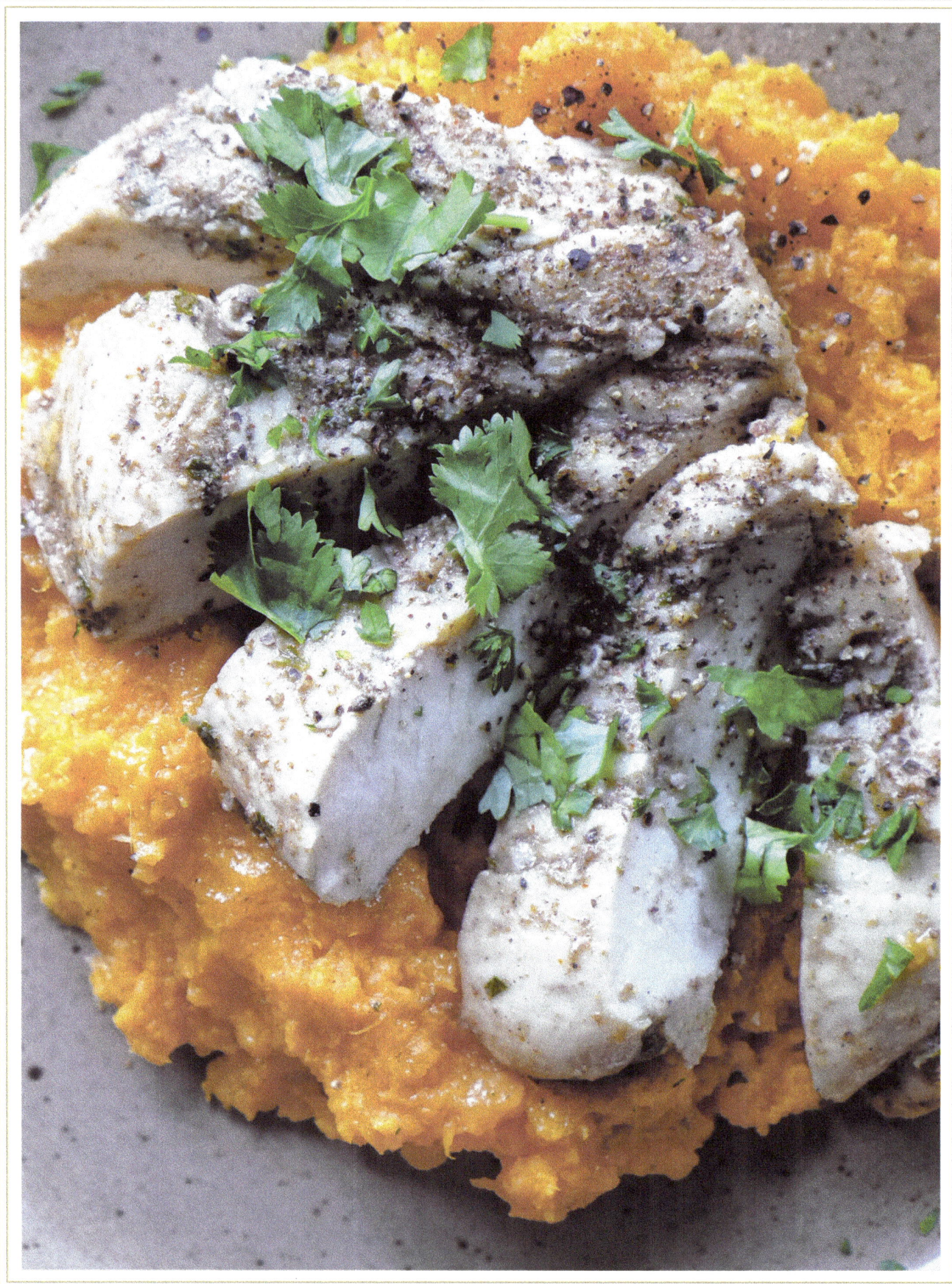

Egyptian Chicken & Sweet Potato Mash

Egyptian Marinade
½ cup chopped yellow onion
¼ cup extra-virgin olive oil
3 garlic cloves, peeled
1 tsp. sea salt
1 tsp. ground cumin
1 tsp. ground coriander
½ tsp. black pepper
¼ tsp. ground cardamom

1 lb. chicken thighs or skinless, boneless chicken breasts (pounded to an even thickness)
2 sweet potatoes
2 Tbsp. honey
½ tsp. cinnamon
sea salt, to taste
chopped cilantro or parsley (to garnish)

1. Marinade: Liquefy the marinade ingredients in a food processor fitted with a standard s-blade. You could also use a blender. Pour it into a resealable plastic bag or container. Add the chicken and coat with the marinade.

Marinate for at least an hour or overnight in the refrigerator.

2. <u>Sweet Potato Mash</u>: Carefully slice the sweet potatoes into large disks or just in half. Boil in a pot of salted water until tender. Drain in a colander. Peel off the skins when cool enough to handle. Mash together with the honey, cinnamon, and sea salt. This can be made in advance, just reheat before serving.

3. Preheat your oven to 400°F. Line a rimmed sheet pan with parchment or use a 9×13-inch baking dish instead. Bring the chicken to room temperature on the counter just before cooking.

4. <u>Roast chicken thighs</u>: 35-40 minutes / boneless chicken breasts: 15-25 minutes or until chicken reaches an internal temperature of 165°F at its thickest part. Cooking time will vary depending on the size and thickness of each piece.

5. Rest for 10 minutes before cutting. Serve Egyptian chicken with sweet potato mash. Garnish with fresh herbs if desired.

Sultan's Apricot Chicken

1 lb. boneless, skinless chicken breasts, diced
1 tsp. baking soda
½ cup dried apricots, chopped
¼ cup raisins
½ cup sliced almonds
1 Tbsp. extra-virgin olive oil
1 medium yellow onion, diced
½ tsp. ground cinnamon
freshly ground black pepper, to taste
sea salt, to taste
½ cup low-sodium chicken stock
2 Tbsp. honey
2 Tbsp. fresh lemon juice
chopped fresh dill (optional)

1. To poach the chicken: First dice into bite-sized pieces, then sprinkle with baking soda. Mix well and set aside for 15 minutes. Thoroughly rinse off the baking soda. Bring a pot of salted water to a boil. Simmer chicken for 3 minutes or until just cooked. Transfer to a clean bowl with a slotted utensil.

2. Place the raisins and apricots into a bowl and cover with boiling water to rehydrate. Drain after 5 minutes.

3. Lightly toast the almonds in a dry wide pan. Remove and set aside.

4. Heat the oil in the same pan. Add the chicken, onions, cinnamon, black pepper, and a good dash of sea salt. Sauté over medium-high heat until the onions are translucent.

5. Stir in the apricots and raisins. Cook for a few minutes. Pour in the chicken stock, honey, and lemon juice. Reduce the heat to medium and simmer for about 5 minutes. Season well with salt and pepper.

6. Sprinkle with sliced almonds and dill if desired. Dill is an unexpected, yet traditional garnish for this dish.

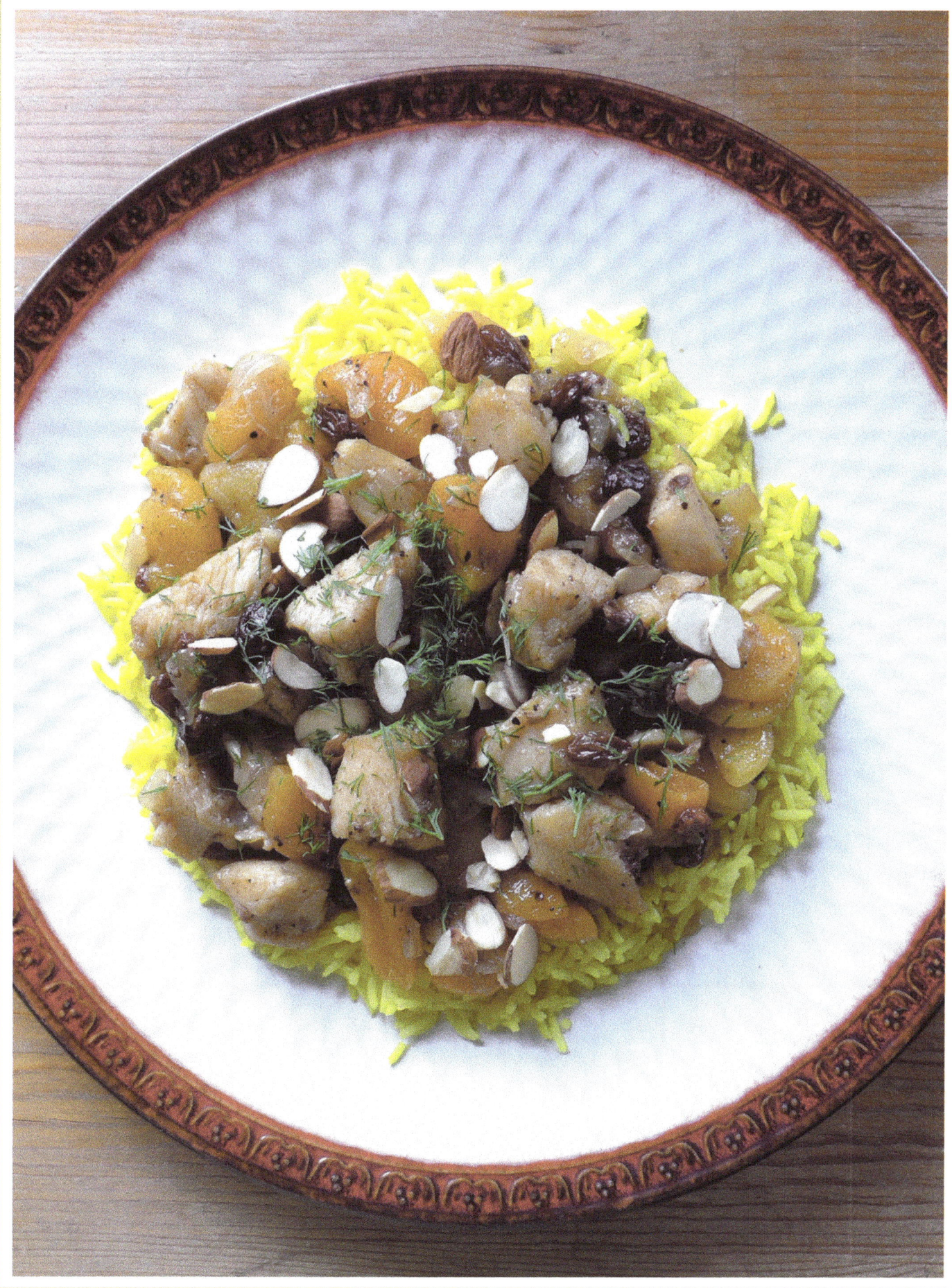

Rosemary & Tomato Braised Chicken

¼ cup tomato paste
1 cup low-sodium chicken stock
6-8 chicken pieces (a combination of chicken thighs and drumsticks)
2 Tbsp. extra-virgin olive oil
sea salt and freshly ground black pepper, to taste
3 garlic cloves, minced
3 rosemary sprigs
pinch red pepper flakes
½ cup white wine
1 cup water, plus more as needed
accompaniment: crusty bread

1. Whisk together the tomato paste and chicken stock in a bowl. Set aside for now.
2. Pat the chicken dry with paper towel. Heat the olive oil in a wide pot with a lid. Arrange the chicken in a single layer. Season with salt and pepper. Brown on all sides, turning occasionally.
3. Lower the heat a bit and add the garlic, rosemary, and red pepper flakes. Cook gently for a few minutes so that the garlic doesn't burn.

4. Pour in the wine to deglaze the pan. Swirl it around and scrape up any bits with a spatula.

5. Pour in the tomato mixture and add a cup of water. Bring to a simmer, then reduce the heat to low. Cover the pot and let the chicken braise for 45 minutes. Flip the chicken pieces every 10-15 minutes. Add a spoonful of water if the sauce starts to dry out. Season with salt and pepper.

6. Serve with roasted potatoes, vegetables, polenta, pasta, spaghetti squash, or just mop up the sauce with some crusty bread.

Chianti Pulled Pork with Tuscan Kale

1 lb. pork tenderloin, loin, or other lean boneless pork, cut into chunks
3 Tbsp. extra-virgin olive oil, divided
¾ tsp. ground fennel (or 1 tsp. fennel seeds, crushed)
sea salt
freshly ground black pepper
pinch red pepper flakes
1 bay leaf
1 Tbsp minced garlic, divided
1 Tbsp. tomato paste
1½ cup Chianti or other red wine
water, as needed
1 bunch Tuscan kale (i.e., cavolo nero, lacinato, black kale)
1 (15-oz.) can cannellini beans, drained and rinsed (optional)

    1. <u>Chianti Pulled Pork</u>: Pat the pork dry and drizzle with a tablespoon of olive oil. Sprinkle the fennel and season well with salt and pepper. Mix well. Heat another tablespoon of the olive oil in a wide pot with a lid. Brown the pork on all sides.

2. Reduce the heat and push the pork to one side. Add a pinch of red pepper flakes, the bay leaf, and two teaspoons of garlic. Cook for 30 seconds. Stir in the tomato paste and let it cook for two minutes.

3. Pour in the wine to deglaze the pot. Swirl it around and scrape up any bits. Release the tomato paste from the bottom and stir it into the mixture.

4. Bring to a boil, then reduce the heat to low. Cover and simmer gently for an hour or until tender. Turn the pieces occasionally. If the pot gets too dry while braising, add a spoonful of water.

5. If the sauce is too thin, remove the lid and boil for a few minutes to thicken. Shred the meat with two forks. Give everything a good stir to mop up the red wine reduction. Season with salt and pepper.

6. <u>For the kale and beans</u>: Wash the kale. Firmly grasp the thick end of each stalk with one hand. Slide off the leafy greens with your other hand. Stack the leaves and cut into ribbons.

7. Heat the remaining olive oil (1 Tbsp.) and garlic (1 tsp.) in another large pan. Cook for 30 seconds, then stir in the cannellini beans if using. Pile on the kale. Stir occasionally and cook until the kale wilts and the beans are warm. Serve with pulled pork.

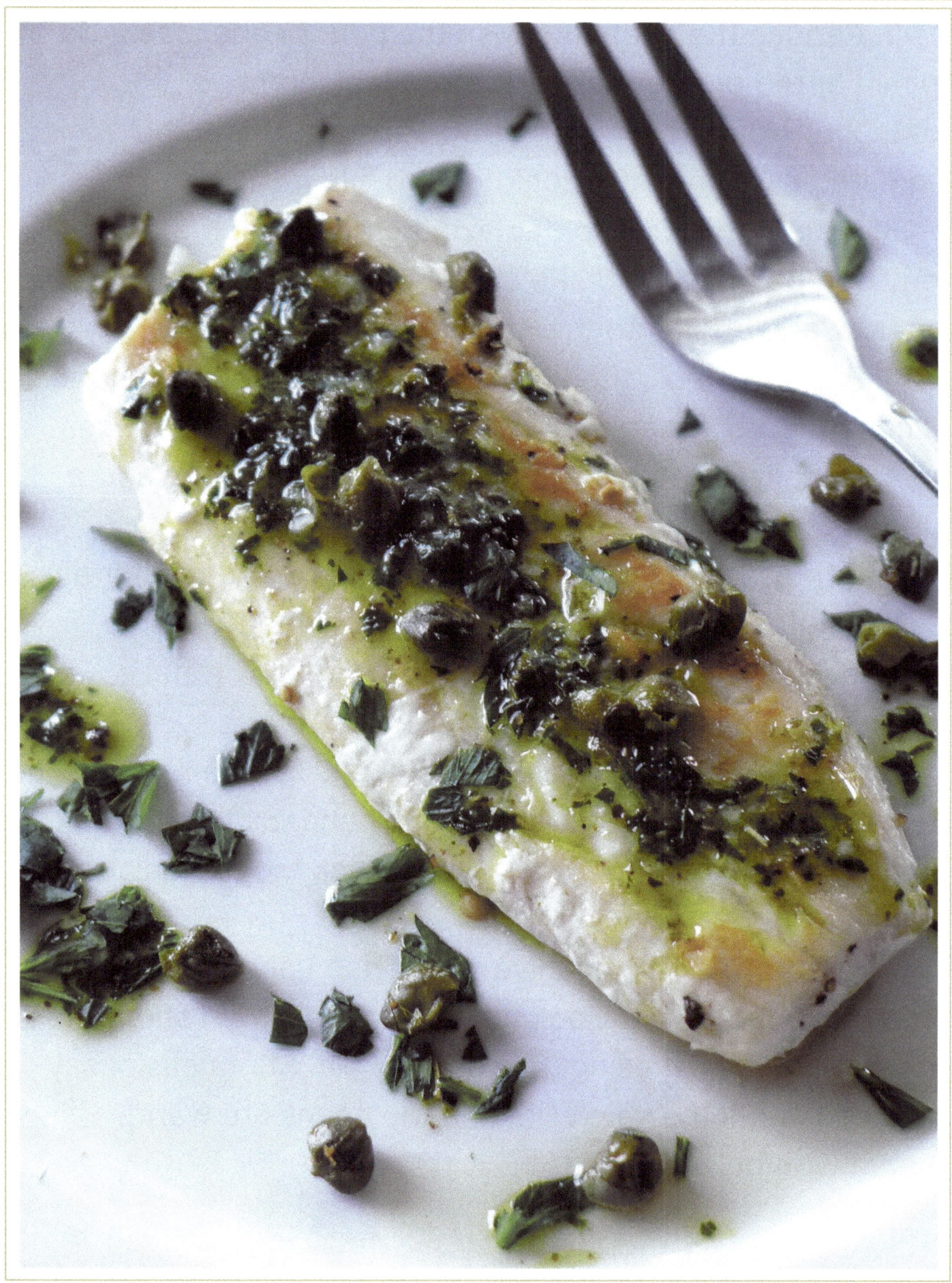

Salmoriglio Skillet Fish

Salmoriglio Sauce
¼ cup extra-virgin olive oil (plus more for the pan)
2 Tbsp. fresh lemon juice
2 Tbsp. flat-leaf parsley leaves, minced
1 tsp. dried oregano
1 garlic clove, minced
½ tsp. sea salt, or more to taste
freshly ground black pepper, to taste

1 lb. white fish fillets (cod, haddock, tilapia, etc.)
2 Tbsp. rinsed capers (optional)

   1. Salmoriglio Sauce: Whisk together the sauce ingredients or use a blender or small food processor. Reserve.
   2. Pat the fish dry with a paper towel. Coat with a small amount of olive oil and season with salt and pepper. Let the fillets come to room temperature before cooking.
   3. Add just a teaspoon of olive oil to a non-stick skillet over medium heat. Cook fillets 2-3 minutes depending on thickness. Flip the fish over and add the capers if using. Cook for another 2-3 minutes or until done to your

preference. Transfer to a clean plate. Spoon some sauce and capers onto the fish.

To use as a marinade: pat fish dry; coat with Salmoriglio; marinate at room temperature for 15 minutes. Immediately grill, bake, or pan-fry as desired.

Baked Chermoula Salmon

Chermoula is a zesty, herbaceous Moroccan sauce often used to marinate fish. Toss a bit with some rice or roasted vegetables for an easy side.

Chermoula
¼ cup extra-virgin olive oil
1 lemon, juice and zest
3 garlic cloves, peeled
1 tsp. ground coriander
½ tsp. ground cumin
¼ tsp. cayenne pepper
¼ tsp. black pepper

1 tsp. fine sea salt
1 cup cilantro with tender stems
1 cup flat-leaf parsley leaves

4 (6-oz.) salmon fillets, skin on

1. <u>Chermoula</u>: Process ingredients in a food processor or finely mince by hand and mix well. Set aside half of the Chermoula to use later as a fresh sauce.

2. <u>To marinate</u>: Place salmon fillets skin-side down into a baking dish. Coat with half of the Chermoula. Cover and refrigerate for at least an hour or overnight if desired.

3. <u>To bake</u>: Preheat your oven to 400°F. Let the salmon come to room temperature on the counter before baking. Bake 11-15 minutes depending on the thickness of your fish. Serve with remaining Chermoula.

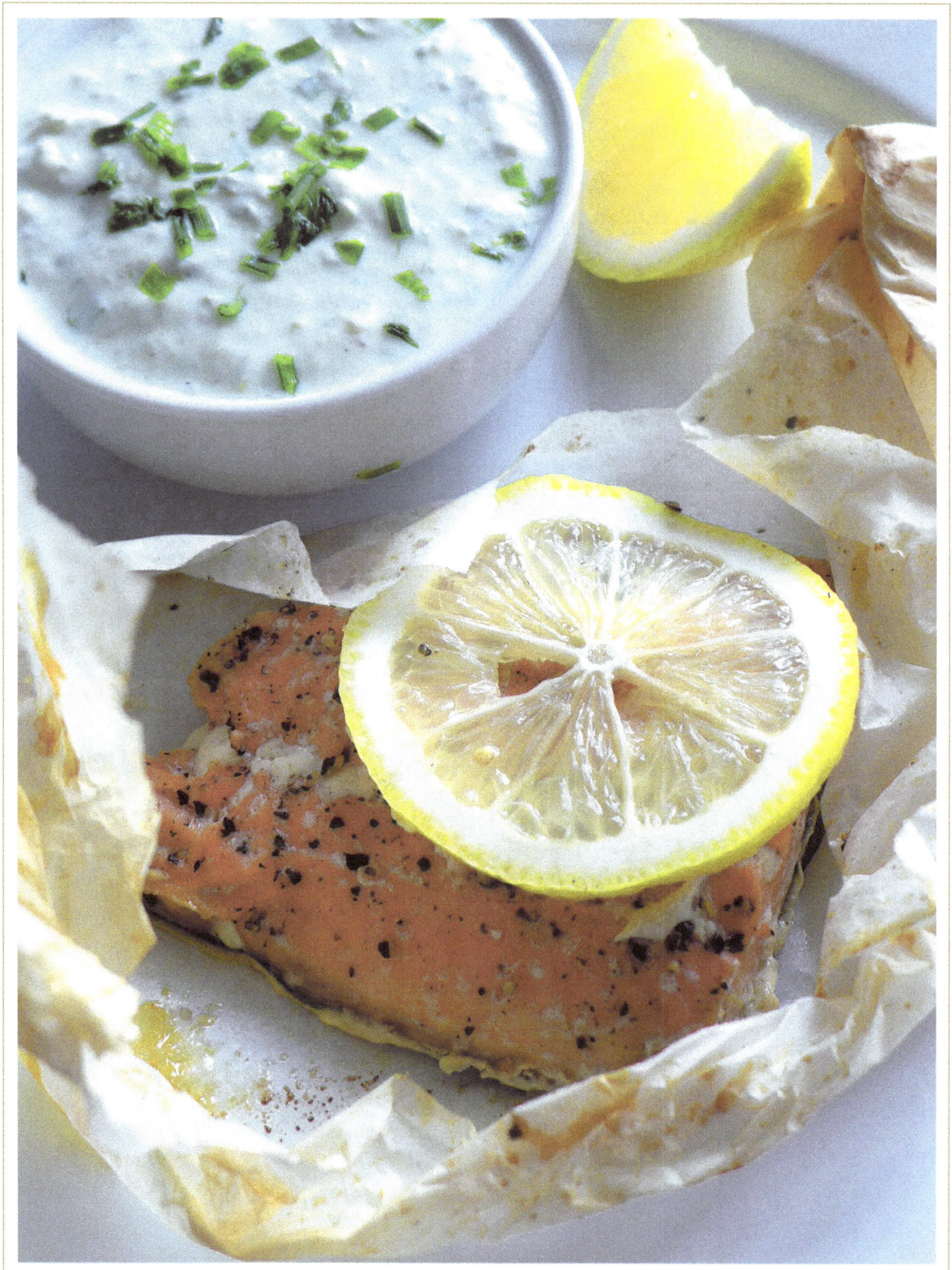

Parchment Baked Salmon with Chive & Horseradish Sauce

This classic French method makes it easy to eat more salmon, one of the most nutrient-dense foods in the world.

Chive & Horseradish Sauce

½ cup Greek yogurt (preferably whole milk) or sour cream
1 to 2 Tbsp. prepared horseradish (squeezed to remove juice)
2 Tbsp. minced chives (plus more to garnish)
1 tsp. fresh lemon juice
sea salt
freshly ground black pepper

4 (6-oz.) salmon fillets
1 Tbsp. extra-virgin olive oil
sea salt and freshly ground black pepper
1 lemon, sliced

Variation

Add a layer of fresh herbs, shredded carrots, asparagus, green beans, or sliced zucchini. Adjust cooking time as needed.

1. <u>Chive & Horseradish Sauce</u>: Squeeze the horseradish to remove juice. Combine with the rest of the ingredients in a small bowl. Mix well and season with salt and pepper. Reserve.

2. <u>For the salmon</u>: Preheat your oven to 400°F. Cut four pieces of parchment large enough to comfortably enclose the fish and whatever else you'd like to add to the packet.

3. Place each fillet (skin-side down if applicable) onto a piece of parchment. Coat with the olive oil and season with salt and pepper. Top with lemon slices.

4. Fold the parchment in half covering each fillet. Starting at one end, crimp overlapping folds along the open side to tightly seal the packets. Place onto a rimmed sheet pan.

5. Bake 10-20 minutes (depending on thickness) or until the internal temperature is 145°F at the thickest parts.

6. Remove the steamed lemon slices if you wish and serve with fresh lemon wheels or wedges instead. Enjoy right away with a dollop of Chive & Horseradish Sauce and a sprinkling of chives.

Hvar Island Fish & Potatoes

This ancient dish is never stirred, but shaken a few times as it simmers. Gregada is one of the oldest ways to prepare fish in Dalmatia and a specialty on the island of Hvar.

½ cup extra-virgin olive oil
1 large onion, diced
3 garlic cloves, minced
sea salt
freshly ground black pepper
1 bay leaf
3 russet potatoes, peeled and sliced into ½-inch rounds
1 lb. firm-fleshed white fish fillets, cut in half if large (or whole fish, cleaned, scaled, and cut into thick pieces)
2 cups white wine
water or fish stock (substitute: a light vegetable or chicken stock)
¼ cup chopped parsley
accompaniments: crusty bread

1. Heat the olive oil in a wide, heavy-bottomed pan. Sauté the onions and garlic until soft. Season with a good pinch of sea salt and black pepper. Add the bay leaf and turn off the heat.

2. Place a layer of potato slices, then top with a layer of fish. Pour in the wine and just enough water or stock to cover. Simmer for about 20 minutes. Never stir, but occasionally shake the pan. Sprinkle with the parsley and season to taste.

3. A shallow bowl is perfect for Gregada. Plate the fish and potatoes with a spoonful of broth. You'll want to clean the plate with a hunk of bread.

Dobar tek!

> "A fish should swim three times...
> in the sea, then in olive oil,
> and finally in wine."
>
> —Croatian expression

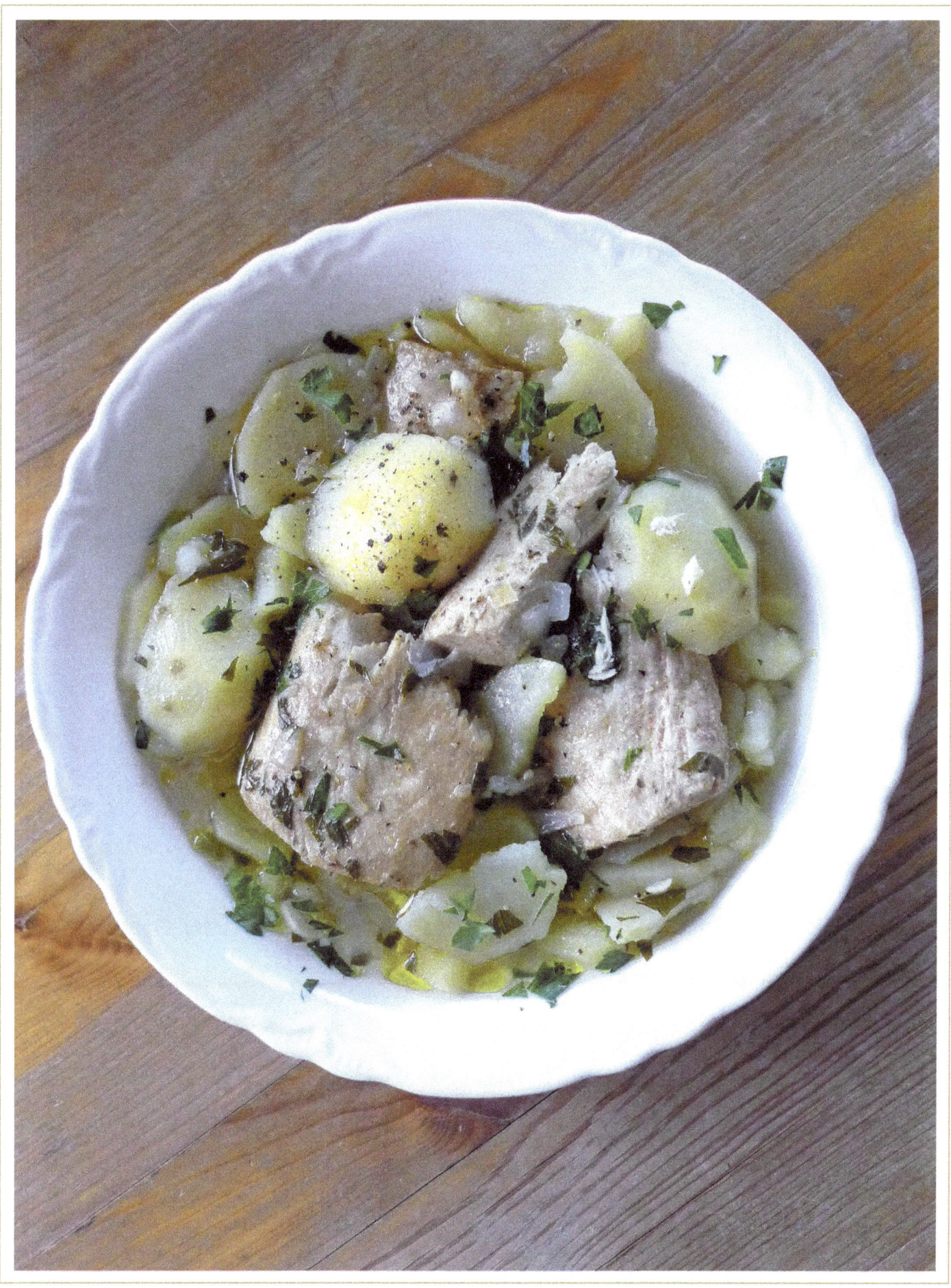

Spicy Braised Fish

¼ cup extra-virgin olive oil
1 onion, diced
1 Tbsp. minced garlic
2 tsp. paprika
1 tsp. cumin
1 tsp. cayenne pepper
½ tsp. red pepper flakes
½ tsp. sea salt
¼ tsp. black pepper
¼ cup tomato paste
1½ cup water
1 lb. white fish fillets (cod, haddock, tilapia, etc.)
1 lemon, cut into wedges
chopped cilantro (garnish)

1. Heat the olive oil in a wide, heavy-bottomed pan. Cook the onions and garlic until soft.
2. Stir in all of the spices and gently cook for about a minute over medium heat. Smash in the tomato paste and cook for a few more minutes. Stir in the water to form a smooth sauce.

3. Place the fillets into the sauce and spoon some over the fish. Bring to a simmer, then reduce the heat to low. Cover the pan and cook for 15 to 20 minutes depending on the thickness of your fillets.

4. Season with sea salt as needed. Sprinkle with cilantro and serve with lemon wedges.

Spanish Garlic Shrimp

1 lb. jumbo shrimp, peeled and deveined
sea salt and freshly ground black pepper
1 tsp. smoked paprika
5 Tbsp. extra-virgin olive oil
5 large garlic cloves, thinly sliced
½ tsp. red pepper flakes (or two dried arbol or japones chiles)
½ cup dry sherry or white wine
¼ cup chopped parsley
traditional accompaniment: toasted bread (to soak up the sauce)

1. Dry the shrimp with paper towel so that it doesn't splatter when added to the hot oil. Season well with sea salt, black pepper, and smoked paprika.

2. Add the garlic and red pepper flakes. Gently cook for about two minutes to infuse the oil with flavor (without browning the garlic).

3. Add the shrimp in a single layer. Flip after about 2 minutes. Pour in the sherry and give the pan a good shake. Increase the heat to medium-high and cook for another minute or two.

4. Pour the shrimp and sauce into a serving dish or terra cotta cazuela. Sprinkle with parsley. Serve with crusty toasted bread to soap up the juices.

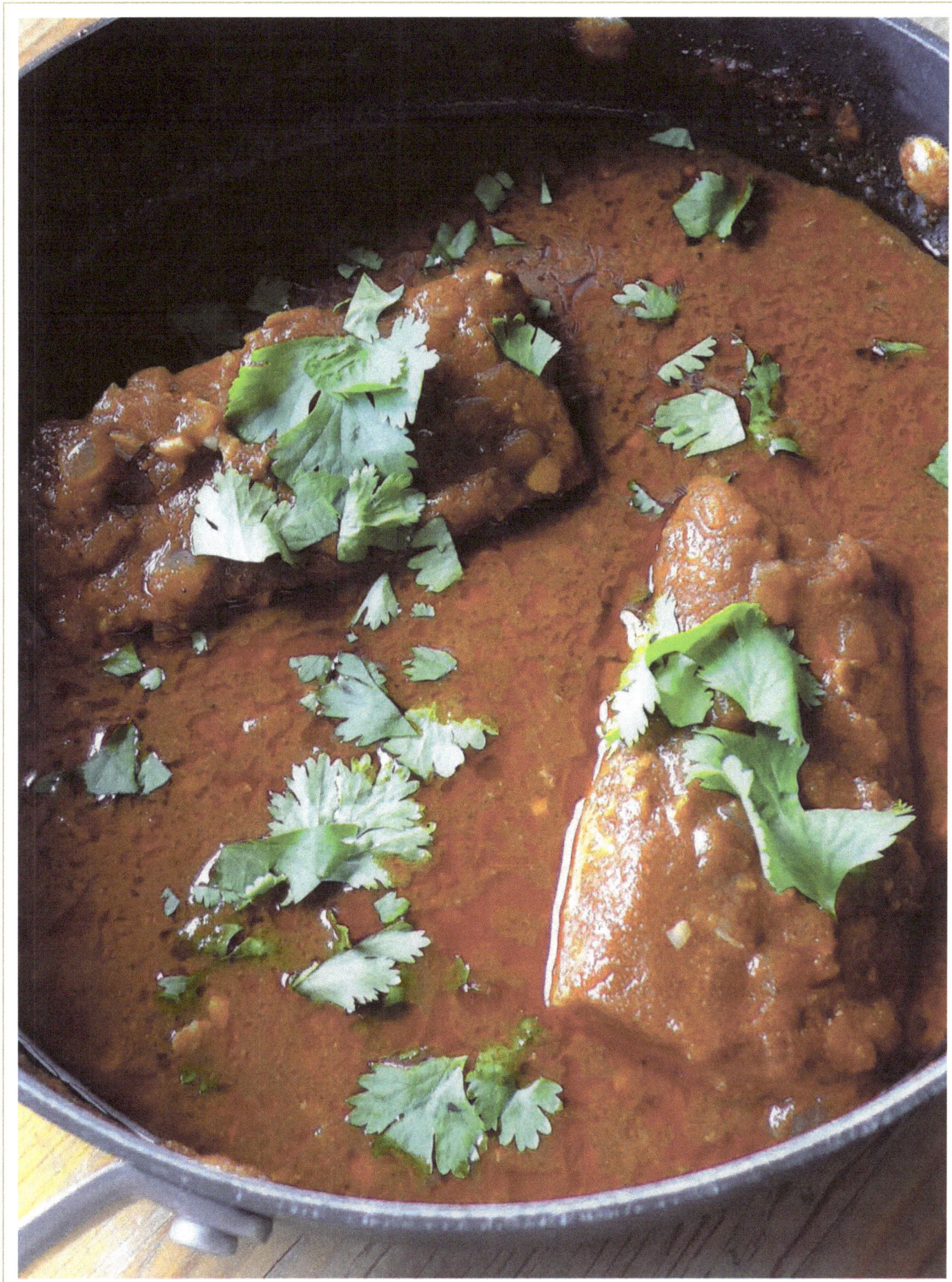

INDEX

#

100% Whole-Wheat Pancakes with Red Wine Blueberry Compote, 39-41

A

Adriatic Herb Chicken, 163-164
Aegean Herb Salad with Greek Feta Dressing, 109-110
Almond(s)
    Apricot, Almond & Dark Chocolate Granola Clusters, 38-39
    Sultan's Apricot Chicken, 169-170
Appetizers, 73
    Feta & Watermelon, 76
    Garden Kebabs, 78
    Greek Meatballs with Feta Mousse, 85-87
    Grilled Prosciutto & Cantaloupe Skewers, 77
    Honey Dill Salmon Brochettes, 82
    Lamb Arrosticini with Mint Gremolata, 81
    Lemon & Spice Pork Pinchitos, 79-80
    Marinated Feta & Olives, 75
    Marinated Mushrooms, 74
    Roasted Cauliflower Bites with Jalapeno Tahini Dip, 83
    Turkish Hot Wings, 84
Apricot(s)
    Apricot, Almond & Dark Chocolate Granola Clusters, 22
    Sultan's Apricot Chicken, 169-170
    Arugula & Parmesan Salad, 107

B

Baked Croutons, 90
Baked Chermoula Salmon, 178-179
Baked Pita Chips, 48
Balela Bean Salad, 99
Balkan Spinach Eggs, 27
Balsamic
    Balsamic Baby Broccoli, 149
    Balsamic Vinaigrette, 104
    Balsamic Baby Broccoli, 149
    Balsamic Vinaigrette, 104
Basil
    Basil Pomodoro, 50
    Provençal Vegetable Soup with Herb Pistou, 127-128

Basil Pomodoro, 50
Beef
   Egyptian Black-Eyed Pea Stew, 137-138
   Greek Meatballs with Feta Mousse, 85-87
Beet Hummus, Pickled, 70
Berries. See also specific berries
   Red Wine Blueberry Compote, 41
   Summer Berry Salad with Balsamic Vinaigrette, 104
Beverages, 6
   Ginger Milk, 6
   Hibiscus Iced Tea, 7
   Salted Yogurt Drink, 9
   Spanish Honey Coffee, 11
   Strawberry Watermelon Quencher, 8
Black Beans. See also Legumes
   Balela Bean Salad, 99
Black-Eyed Peas. See also Legumes
   Black-Eyed Pea Tuna Salad, 103
   Egyptian Black-Eyed Pea Stew, 137-138
Braised
   Chianti Pulled Pork with Tuscan Kale, 174-175
   Rosemary & Tomato Braised Chicken, 172-173
   Spicy Braised Fish, 186-187
Breakfast, 13
   100% Whole-Wheat Pancakes with Red Wine Blueberry Compote, 39-40
   Apricot, Almond & Dark Chocolate Granola Clusters, 22
   Balkan Spinach Eggs, 27
   Catalan Tomato Toast, 20
   Good Morning Graze, 14
   Greek Yogurt with Roasted Strawberries, 16
   Istrian Wild Asparagus Fritaja, 25
   Labneh Yogurt Spread, 17
   Milk & Honey Barley Porridge, 42
   Olive Oil-Basted Eggs, 21
   Portobello Baked Eggs, 29
   Quick & Cold Bulgur Cereal, 37
   Spanish Zucchini Scramble, 23
   Strained Yogurt with Honey & Walnuts, 15
   Tahini Honey Butter, 18
   Tomato Harvest Scramble, 22
   Tunisian Protein Bowl with Harissa, 31-33
   Turkish Poached Eggs with Feta-Yogurt Sauce, 33-34
Broccoli, Balsamic, 149

Brochettes. See Skewers

Bruschetta
- Garlic Bruschetta Toast, 47

Brussels Sprouts, Roasted, 148

Bulgur
- Quick & Cold Bulgur Cereal, 37
- Tomato Bulgur Pilaf, 157

C

Cannellini Tuna Salad with Fried Capers, 100-101

Capers
- Fried Capers, 100-101
- Salmoriglio Skillet Fish, 177-178
- Tunisian Protein Bowl with Harissa, 31-33

Carrot(s)
- Roasted Jalapeno Carrot Dip, 59

Catalan Tomato Toast, 11

Cauliflower
- Roasted Cauliflower Bites with Jalapeno Tahini Dip, 83

Chermoula, Baked Salmon, 178-179

Chianti Pulled Pork with Tuscan Kale, 174-175

Chocolate
- Apricot, Almond & Dark Chocolate Granola Clusters, 22

Chicken
- Adriatic Herb Chicken, 163-164
- Egyptian Chicken with Sweet Potato Mash, 167-168
- Italian Chicken Sub Salad, 105-106
- Rosemary & Tomato Braised Chicken, 172-173
- Salad Bar Chicken, 94-95
- Sultan's Apricot Chicken, 169-170
- Turkish Hot Wings, 84
- White Chicken Noodle Soup, 132-133

Chickpeas. See also legumes, Hummus
- Balela Bean Salad, 99
- Sea Salt Roasted Chickpeas, 92
- Tunisian Protein Bowl with Harissa, 31-33
- White Chicken Noodle Soup, 132-133

Chive & Horseradish Sauce, 181-182

Cilantro
- Cilantro Rice, 155
- Lemon & Cilantro Lentil Soup, 119-120

Zhoug Hot Sauce, 52
Cilantro Rice, 155
Classic Hummus, 68
Coffee, Spanish Honey, 6
Croatian
- Dalmatian Chard & Potatoes, 145
- Hvar Island Fish & Potatoes, 183-184
- Istrian Wild Asparagus Fritaja, 25

Crostini Bites, 46
Cucumber(s)
- Cucumber Tzatziki, 56
- Egyptian Smashed Feta & Cucumber Salad, 96
- Moroccan Tomato & Cucumber Salad, 97
- Cucumber Tzatziki, 56

D

Dalmatian Chard & Potatoes, 145
Dill
- Dill Hot Sauce, 123
- Honey Dill Salmon Brochettes, 82

Dips (and Spreads), 44. See also Hummus
- Chive & Horseradish Sauce, 181-182
- Eggplant Mutabal, 58
- Feta Mousse, 85-87
- Jalapeno Tahini Dip, 83
- Labneh Yogurt Spread, 17
- Mandarin Fig Jam, 55
- Olive Spread, 53
- Onion Marmalade, 54
- Roasted Jalapeno Carrot Dip, 59
- Santorini Yellow Pea Dip, 62-63
- Spicy Whipped Feta Dip, 57
- Tahini Honey Butter, 18
- Tomato Matbucha, 60-61
- Tuscan Dipping Oil, 49

Dressings
- Balsamic Vinaigrette, 104
- Greek Feta Dressing, 109
- Old Style Mustard Vinaigrette, 112-113
- Sub Sauce, Italian, 105

E

Eggplant
- Eggplant Mutabal, 58
- Greek Vegetable Bake, 162-163
- Roasted Eggplant Cubes, 93
- Eggplant Mutabal, 58

Eggs
- Balkan Spinach Eggs, 27
- Istrian Wild Asparagus Fritaja, 25

Olive Oil-Basted Eggs, 21
Portobello Baked Eggs, 29
Spanish Zucchini Scramble, 23
Tomato Harvest Scramble, 22
Turkish Poached Eggs with Feta-Yogurt Sauce, 33-34
Tunisian Protein Bowl with Harissa, 31-33
Egyptian Black-Eyed Pea Stew, 137-138
Egyptian
- Egyptian Black-Eyed Pea Stew, 137-138
- Egyptian Chicken with Sweet Potato Mash, 167-168
- Egyptian Smashed Feta & Cucumber Salad, 96
- Hibiscus Iced Tea, 5

Egyptian Chicken with Sweet Potato Mash, 167-168
Egyptian Smashed Feta & Cucumber Salad, 96

F

Feta & Watermelon, 76
Feta Cheese
- Egyptian Smashed Feta & Cucumber Salad, 96
- Feta & Watermelon, 76
- Greek Feta Dressing, 109
- Greek Meatballs with Feta Mousse, 85-87
- Marinated Feta & Olives, 75
- Spicy Whipped Feta Dip, 57
- Turkish Poached Eggs with Feta-Yogurt Sauce, 33-34

Feta Mousse, 85-87
Fig
- Mandarin Fig Jam, 55

Fish
- Baked Chermoula Salmon, 178-179
- Hvar Island Fish & Potatoes, 183-184
- Maltese Fish Soup, 138-139
- Parchment Baked Salmon with Chive & Horseradish Sauce, 181-182
- Salmoriglio Skillet Fish, 177-178
- Spicy Braised Fish, 186-187

French
- Honey Dill Salmon Brochettes, 82
- Mushroom Duxelles Brown Rice, 158
- Onion Marmalade, 54
- Parchment Baked Salmon with Chive & Horseradish Sauce, 181-182
- Poached Salmon Niçoise with Old Style Mustard Vinaigrette, 112-114

Provençal Vegetable Soup with Herb Pistou, 127-128
Roasted Mushrooms Persillade, 147
Fried
   Capers, 53
   Sage, 70
   Salmoriglio Skillet Fish, 177-178
Fruit. See also specific fruit
   Greek Yogurt with Roasted Strawberries, 16
   100% Whole-Wheat Pancakes with Red Wine Blueberry Compote, 39-40
   Mandarin Fig Jam, 55
   Greek Yogurt with Roasted Strawberries, 16
   Strawberry Watermelon Quencher, 8
   Sultan's Apricot Chicken, 169-170

G

Garden Kebabs, 78
Garlic
   Dalmatian Chard & Potatoes, 145
   Garlic Bruschetta Toast, 47
   Roasted Garlic Hummus, 72
   Spanish Garlic Shrimp, 187-188
   Garlic Bruschetta Toast, 47
Ginger Milk, 10
Good Morning Graze, 14
Grains
   100% Whole-Wheat Pancakes with Red Wine Blueberry Compote, 39-40
   Apricot, Almond & Dark Chocolate Granola Clusters, 22
   Milk & Honey Barley Porridge, 42
   Quick & Cold Bulgur Cereal, 37
   Whole Grain Tabouli, 98
Granola, Apricot, Almond & Dark Chocolate Clusters, 38
Greek
   Aegean Herb Salad with Greek Feta Dressing, 109-110
   Baked Pita Chips, 48
   Cucumber Tzatziki, 56
   Feta Mousse, 85-87
   Greek Dandelion Greens, 144
   Greek Feta Dressing, 109
   Greek Meatballs with Feta Mousse, 85-87
   Greek Pork & Celery Stew, 129-130
   Greek Salsa, 51
   Greek Vegetable Bake, 162-

163
- Santorini Yellow Pea Dip, 62-63
- Spicy Whipped Feta Dip, 57
- Spinach Rice, 154
- Stewed Green Beans, 151-152
- Tahini Honey Butter, 18
- Tomato Harvest Scramble, 22

Greek Feta Dressing, 109
Greek Meatballs with Feta Mousse, 85-87
Greek Pork & Celery Stew, 129-130
Greek Vegetable Bake, 162-163
Greek Yogurt with Roasted Strawberries, 16
Greens
- Balkan Spinach Eggs, 27
- Chianti Pulled Pork with Tuscan Kale, 174-175
- Dalmatian Chard & Potatoes, 145
- Greek Dandelion Greens, 144
- Greek Pork & Celery Stew, 129-130
- Lemon & Cilantro Lentil Soup, 119-120
- Spinach Rice, 154

Green Beans, Stewed, 151-152
Gremolata, Mint, 44
Grilled Prosciutto & Cantaloupe Skewers, 77

H

Harissa, 32
Hibiscus Iced Tea, 5
Honey
- Honey Dill Salmon Brochettes, 82
- Honey Roasted Nuts, 91
- Spanish Honey Coffee, 11
- Strained Yogurt with Honey & Walnuts, 15
- Sultan's Apricot Chicken, 169-170
- Tahini Honey Butter, 18

Honey Dill Salmon Brochettes, 82
Honey Roasted Nuts, 91
Hot Sauces
- Dill Hot Sauce, 123
- Harissa, 32
- Zhoug Hot Sauce, 52

Hummus, 66-72
- Black Olive Hummus, 69
- Classic Hummus, 68
- Jalapeno Hummus, 71
- Pickled Beet Hummus, 70
- Red Pepper Hummus, 69
- Roasted Garlic Hummus, 72

Hvar Island Fish & Potatoes, 183-184

I

Istrian Wild Asparagus Fritaja, 25

Italian
- Arugula & Parmesan Salad, 107
- Basil Pomodoro, 50
- Cannellini Tuna Salad with Fried Capers, 100-101
- Chianti Pulled Pork with Tuscan Kale, 174-175
- Garlic Bruschetta Toast, 47
- Grilled Prosciutto & Cantaloupe Skewers, 77
- Italian Chicken Sub Salad, 105-106
- Lamb Arrosticini with Mint Gremolata, 81
- Marinated Mushrooms, 74
- Rosemary & Tomato Braised Chicken, 172-173
- Salmoriglio Skillet Fish, 177-178
- Tuscan Dipping Oil, 49

Italian Chicken Sub Salad, 105-106

J

Jalapeno
- Jalapeno Hummus, 71
- Roasted Cauliflower Bites with Jalapeno Tahini Dip, 83
- Roasted Jalapeno Carrot Dip, 59
- Jalapeno Tahini Dip, 83
- Jalapeno Hummus, 71

K

Kebabs. See Skewers

Kale, Tuscan
- Chianti Pulled Pork with Tuscan Kale, 174-175
- Greek Pork & Celery Stew, 129-130

L

Labneh Yogurt Spread, 17

Lamb Arrosticini with Mint Gremolata, 81

Lamb
- Lamb Arrosticini with Mint Gremolata, 81
- Libyan Minted Lamb Soup, 135-136

Legumes. See also specific varieties
- Balela Bean Salad, 99
- Chianti Pulled Pork with

Tuscan Kale, 174-175

   Greek Pork & Celery Stew, 129-130
   Lemon & Cilantro Lentil Soup, 119-120
   Libyan Minted Lamb Soup, 135-136
   Mujadara Lentil Dip, 63-64
   Red Lentil Soup with Dill Hot Sauce, 122-123
   Santorini Yellow Pea Dip, 62-63
   Sea Salt Roasted Chickpeas, 92
   Tunisian Protein Bowl with Harissa, 31-33
   White Chicken Noodle Soup, 132-133

Lemon & Cilantro Lentil Soup, 119-120

Lemon & Spice Pork Pinchitos, 79-80

Lentils. See also Legumes
   Mujadara Lentil Dip, 63-64
   Red Lentil Soup with Dill Hot Sauce, 122-123
   Libyan Minted Lamb Soup, 135-136

M

Mains, 161
   Adriatic Herb Chicken, 163-164
   Baked Chermoula Salmon, 178-179
   Chianti Pulled Pork with Tuscan Kale, 174-175
   Egyptian Chicken with Sweet Potato Mash, 167-168
   Greek Vegetable Bake, 162-163
   Hvar Island Fish & Potatoes, 183-184
   Parchment Baked Salmon with Chive & Horseradish Sauce, 181-182
   Rosemary & Tomato Braised Chicken, 172-173
   Salmoriglio Skillet Fish, 177-178
   Spanish Garlic Shrimp, 187-188
   Spicy Braised Fish, 186-187
   Sultan's Apricot Chicken, 169-170

Maltese Fish Soup, 138-139

Mandarin Fig Jam, 55

Meatballs, Greek with Feta Mousse, 85-87

Melon, See also Watermelon
   Feta & Watermelon, 76

Grilled Prosciutto & Cantaloupe Skewers, 77
Strawberry Watermelon Quencher, 8

Middle Eastern
- Balela Bean Salad, 99
- Eggplant Mutabal, 58
- Feta & Watermelon, 76
- Ginger Milk, 10
- Hummus, 66-72
- Labneh Yogurt Spread, 17
- Lemon & Cilantro Lentil Soup, 119-120
- Mujadara Lentil Dip, 63-64
- Orange Soup with Fried Sage, 125-126
- Roasted Cauliflower Bites with Jalapeno Tahini Dip, 83
- Roasted Jalapeno Carrot Dip, 59
- Stewed Green Beans, 151-152
- Whole Grain Tabouli, 98
- Yellow Rice Pilaf, 156

Milk & Honey Barley Porridge, 42

Mint
- Lamb Arrosticini with Mint Gremolata, 81
- Libyan Minted Lamb Soup, 135-136
- Whole Grain Tabouli, 98

Mint Gremolata, 44

Moroccan
- Baked Chermoula Salmon, 178-179
- Moroccan Tomato & Cucumber Salad, 51
- Spicy Braised Fish, 186-187
- Tomato Matbucha, 60-61

Moroccan Tomato & Cucumber Salad, 97

Mujadara Lentil Dip, 63-64

Mushroom Duxelles Brown Rice, 158

Mushroom(s)
- Marinated Mushrooms, 74
- Mushroom Duxelles Brown Rice, 158
- Portobello Baked Eggs, 29
- Roasted Mushrooms Persillade, 147

Mustard Vinaigrette, Old Style, 112-113

N

Niçoise, Poached Salmon, 112-114

North African. See also specific cuisines
- Baked Chermoula Salmon, 178-179

Egyptian Black-Eyed Pea Stew, 137-138
Egyptian Chicken with Sweet Potato Mash, 167-168

Egyptian Smashed Feta & Cucumber Salad, 96
Hibiscus Iced Tea, 5
Libyan Minted Lamb Soup, 135-136
Moroccan Tomato & Cucumber Salad, 97
Spicy Braised Fish, 186-187
Tomato Matbucha, 60-61
Tunisian Protein Bowl with Harissa, 31-33
White Chicken Noodle Soup, 132-133

O

Old Style Mustard Vinaigrette, 112-113
Olives
   Black Olive Hummus, 69
   Marinated Feta & Olives, 75
   Olive Spread, 53
   Olive Oil-Basted Eggs, 21
Olive Spread, 53
Onion Marmalade, 54
Orange Soup with Fried Sage, 125-126

P

Parchment Baked Salmon with Chive & Horseradish Sauce, 181-182
Parsley
   Aegean Herb Salad with Greek Feta Dressing, 109-110
   Roasted Mushrooms Persillade, 147
   Whole Grain Tabouli, 98
   Persillade, Mushrooms, 147
Pickled Beet Hummus, 70
Pita Chips, Baked, 48
Pinchitos, Lemon & Spice Pork, 79-80
Pork
   Chianti Pulled Pork with Tuscan Kale, 174-175
   Greek Pork & Celery Stew, 129-130
   Lemon & Spice Pork Pinchitos, 79-80
Portobello Baked Eggs, 29
Potatoes
   Dalmatian Chard & Potatoes, 145
   Hvar Island Fish & Potatoes, 183-184
   Salmon Pot, 140-141

Prosciutto
   Grilled Prosciutto & Cantaloupe Skewers, 77
Provençal Vegetable Soup with Herb Pistou, 127-128

Q

Quick & Cold Bulgur Cereal, 37

R

Red Lentil Soup with Dill Hot Sauce, 122-123
Red Pepper Hummus, 69
Red Wine Blueberry Compote, 41
Rice
   Cilantro Rice, 155
   Maltese Fish Soup, 138-139
   Mushroom Duxelles Brown Rice, 158
   Spinach Rice, 154
   Yellow Rice Pilaf, 156
Roasted Brussels Sprouts, 148
Roasted Cauliflower Bites with Jalapeno Tahini Dip, 83
Roasted Eggplant Cubes, 93
Roasted Garlic Hummus, 72
Roasted Jalapeno Carrot Dip, 59
Roasted Mushrooms Persillade, 147
Roasted Spaghetti Squash, 159
Rosemary & Tomato Braised Chicken, 172-173

S

Salad Bar Chicken, 94-95
Salads, 89
   Aegean Herb Salad with Greek Feta Dressing, 109-110
   Arugula & Parmesan Salad, 107
   Balela Bean Salad, 99
   Black-Eyed Pea Tuna Salad, 103
   Cannellini Tuna Salad with Fried Capers, 100-101
   Egyptian Smashed Feta & Cucumber Salad, 96
   Italian Chicken Sub Salad, 105-106
   Moroccan Tomato & Cucumber Salad, 97
   Poached Salmon Niçoise with Old Style Mustard Vinaigrette, 112-114
   Summer Berry Salad with Balsamic Vinaigrette, 104
   Valencian Salad, 110-111

Whole Grain Tabouli, 98
Salmon
   Baked Chermoula Salmon, 178-179
   Honey Dill Salmon Brochettes, 82
   Parchment Baked Salmon with Chive & Horseradish Sauce, 181-182
   Poached Salmon Niçoise with Old Style Mustard Vinaigrette, 112-114
   Salmon Pot, 140-141
   Simple Flaked Salmon, 95-96
Salmon Pot, 140-141
Salmoriglio Skillet Fish, 177-178
Salted Yogurt Drink, 5
Santorini Yellow Pea Dip, 62-63
Scrambled Eggs
   Istrian Wild Asparagus Fritaja, 25
   Spanish Zucchini Scramble, 23
   Tomato Harvest Scramble, 22
Sea Salt Roasted Chickpeas, 92
Shrimp, Spanish Garlic, 187-188
Sides, 143
   Balsamic Baby Broccoli, 149
   Cilantro Rice, 155
   Dalmatian Chard & Potatoes, 145
   Greek Dandelion Greens, 144
   Mushroom Duxelles Brown Rice, 158
   Roasted Brussels Sprouts, 148
   Roasted Mushrooms Persillade, 147
   Roasted Spaghetti Squash, 159
   Spinach Rice, 154
   Stewed Green Beans, 151-152
   Stewed Sweet Peppers, 150-151
   Sweet Potato Mash, 167-168
   Tomato Bulgur Pilaf, 157
   Yellow Rice Pilaf, 156
   Simple Flaked Salmon, 95-96
Skewers
   Garden Kebabs, 78
   Grilled Prosciutto & Cantaloupe Skewers, 77
   Honey Dill Salmon Brochettes, 82
   Lamb Arrosticini with Mint Gremolata, 81
   Lemon & Spice Pork Pinchitos, 79-80
Soups, 117
   Egyptian Black-Eyed Pea Stew, 137-138
   Greek Pork & Celery Stew, 129-130

Lemon & Cilantro Lentil Soup, 119-120
Libyan Minted Lamb Soup, 135-136
Maltese Fish Soup, 138-139
Orange Soup with Fried Sage, 125-126
Provençal Vegetable Soup with Herb Pistou, 127-128
Red Lentil Soup with Dill Hot Sauce, 122-123
Salmon Pot, 140-141
Tunisian Protein Bowl with Harissa, 31-33
White Chicken Noodle Soup, 132-133

Spanish
- Catalan Tomato Toast, 20
- Olive Oil-Basted Eggs, 21
- Spanish Garlic Shrimp, 187-188
- Spanish Honey Coffee, 11
- Spanish Zucchini Scramble, 23
- Valencian Salad, 110-111
- Spanish Garlic Shrimp, 187-188

Spanish Honey Coffee, 11
Spanish Zucchini Scramble, 23

Spicy
- Dill Hot Sauce, 123
- Spanish Garlic Shrimp, 187-188
- Spicy Braised Fish, 186-187
- Spicy Whipped Feta Dip, 57
- Tomato Matbucha, 60-61
- Tunisian Protein Bowl with Harissa, 31-33
- Turkish Hot Wings, 84
- Zhoug Hot Sauce, 52
- Spicy Braised Fish, 186-187
- Spicy Whipped Feta Dip, 57

Spinach
- Balkan Spinach Eggs, 27
- Spinach Rice, 154
- Spinach Rice, 154

Stews. See Soups
Stewed Green Beans, 151-152
Stewed Sweet Peppers, 150-151

Strawberries
- Greek Yogurt with Roasted Strawberries, 16
- Strawberry Watermelon Quencher, 8
- Summer Berry Salad with Balsamic Vinaigrette, 104

Sub Sauce, Italian, 105
Sultan's Apricot Chicken, 169-170
Summer Berry Salad with Balsamic Vinaigrette, 104

Squash. See also specific squash
- Orange Soup with Fried Sage, 125-126

Roasted Spaghetti Squash, 159
Spanish Zucchini Scramble, 23
Sweet Potato Mash, 167-168

T

Tahini
    Roasted Cauliflower Bites with Jalapeno Tahini Dip, 83
    Tahini Honey Butter, 18
Tahini Honey Butter, 18
Tea
    Hibiscus Iced Tea, 5
Toasted
    Baked Croutons, 90
    Baked Pita Chips, 48
    Crostini Bites, 46
    Garlic Bruschetta Toast, 47
Tomato
    Basil Pomodoro, 50
    Catalan Tomato Toast, 20
    Moroccan Tomato & Cucumber Salad, 97
    Rosemary & Tomato Braised Chicken, 172-173
    Tomato Bulgur Pilaf, 157
    Tomato Harvest Scramble, 22
    Tomato Matbucha, 60-61
    Tomato Bulgur Pilaf, 157
    Tomato Matbucha, 60-61
Toppings
    Basil Pomodoro, 50
    Dill Hot Sauce, 123
    Greek Salsa, 51
    Herb Pistou, 127-128
    Zhoug Hot Sauce, 52
Tuna
    Black-Eyed Pea Tuna Salad, 103
    Cannellini Tuna Salad with Fried Capers, 100-101
    Tunisian Protein Bowl with Harissa, 31-33
    Valencian Salad, 110-111
Turkish
    Salted Yogurt Drink, 5
    Sultan's Apricot Chicken, 169-170
    Tomato Bulgur Pilaf, 157
    Turkish Hot Wings, 84
    Turkish Poached Eggs with Feta-Yogurt Sauce, 33-34
Tuscan Dipping Oil, 49
Tzatziki, Cucumber, 56

V

Valencian Salad, 110-111
Vegetable Soup, Provencal, 71
Vinaigrette. See Dressings

W

Walnuts
  Strained Yogurt with Honey & Walnuts, 15
Watermelon
  Feta & Watermelon, 76
  Strawberry Watermelon Quencher, 8
White Chicken Noodle Soup, 132-133
Whole Grain Tabouli, 98
Wine
  Chianti Pulled Pork with Tuscan Kale, 174-175
  Hvar Island Fish & Potatoes, 183-184
  Red Wine Blueberry Compote, 41
  Rosemary & Tomato Braised Chicken, 172-173
  Spanish Garlic Shrimp, 187-188

Y

Yellow Rice Pilaf, 156
Yogurt
  Cucumber Tzatziki, 56
  Greek Yogurt with Roasted Strawberries, 16
  Labneh Yogurt Spread, 17
  Salted Yogurt Drink, 5
  Strained Yogurt with Honey & Walnuts, 15

Z

Zucchini
  Greek Vegetable Bake, 162-163
  Provençal Vegetable Soup with Herb Pistou, 127-128
  Spanish Zucchini Scramble, 23
Greek Vegetable Bake, 162-163
Spanish Zucchini Scramble, 23

www.ingramcontent.com/pod-product-compliance
Lightning Source LLC
Chambersburg PA
CBHW061141010526
44118CB00026B/2841